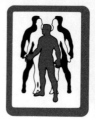

Allied Health Series

Management Procedures

Robert F. Comte, M.T. (AMT)

Leslie W. Lee, M.T. (ASCP)

Consultant/Reviewer

M. Ruth Williams, M.T.

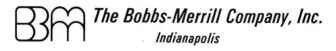 *The Bobbs-Merrill Company, Inc.*
Indianapolis

FIRST EDITION

FIRST PRINTING—1975

The Bobbs-Merrill Company, Inc.
4300 West 62nd Street
Indianapolis, Indiana 46268

Library of Congress Catalog Card Number: 74-18677
ISBN: 0-672-61397-2

Preface

One of the most important developments in the health field in recent years has been the rise of allied health personnel. These persons provide essential services and support for physicians and dentists (including those engaged in specialized practices in these professions) as well as for others engaged in health-oriented fields, such as dental assistants, inhalation therapists, physical therapists, and medical records technicians.

Professional Needs

The day when the physician, in or out of the hospital environment, was able to carry the whole burden of patient care with no help other than that of a nurse is over. Today, the professional nurse herself needs well-trained assistants, and it is generally accepted that health care is a team operation, with the physician as the head of the team. Furthermore, each member of the team must be a skilled technician—able to carry out the increasingly complex techniques required by modern medical care.

Educational Needs

The pressing need for well-trained personnel prepared to serve in the various allied health occupations has opened a whole new field of education. It is no longer possible for a person interested in working as a technician in a medical, dental, or x-ray laboratory to acquire mastery of his chosen field by learning on the job. Although on-the-job training remains important, basic training in the classroom must precede it. This fact has become so evident that schools, laboratories, and hospitals and allied institutions have begun to step up their educational programs to meet the growing demand for trained personnel. Another factor that emphasizes the urgent need for academic training in the allied health fields is the demand by federal, state, and municipal regulatory agencies for the certification and licensing of personnel in an increasing number of these occupational fields.

Educators attempting to respond to the challenge of providing sound educational systems for developing personnel for these jobs found themselves handicapped by the lack of authoritative textbooks that met the special requirements of their students. Students interested in preparing themselves to fill these jobs found it difficult to obtain clear, concise information that was relevant. Persons already employed in allied health fields found it difficult to obtain the additional information they needed to augment and supplement their knowledge and experience.

In response to all of these needs, the Allied Health Occupations Series was conceived. The Series consists of textbooks, workbooks, audio tapes, laboratory manuals, and teacher's guides to provide a wide range of educational materials tailored to meet a variety of requirements and to serve students with various abilities.

About the Allied Health Occupations Series

The Allied Health Occupations Series is especially structured to offer a wide variety of basic tools for creative teaching and learning. Each component of the Series presents detailed, comprehensive information that is easy to read, easy to use, and up to date. All are specifically designed for maximum use by educators, students, and personnel in allied health occupations.

The modularized approach of the Series is unique. It allows unlimited flexibility for the teacher and for the student. The illustration on this page gives a few examples of the multiple use that can be made of materials because of the variance and overlap of informational needs in various allied health fields. Core materials (e.g., *Basic Chemistry* and *Basic Microbiology*) provide basic information; supplementary materials (e.g., *Organic Chemistry* and *Introduction to Diagnostic Microbiology*) provide specific and detailed information. Teachers and students can adapt the materials to meet their special needs.

The books have been carefully designed to invite learning and to aid teaching. Teachers will immediately notice the blocks of text material uninterrupted by hard-to-read italics or boldface type so popular in older textbooks where it was believed necessary to indicate "important" words or phrases. Such artificial techniques are unnecessary in these texts because each has been written to include only that information essential to a

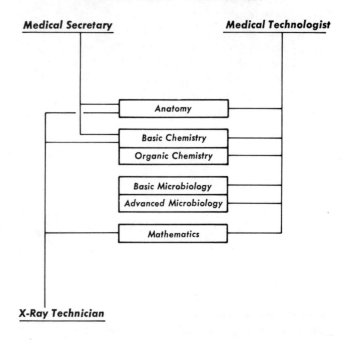

thorough understanding of the subject. Extraneous materials have been removed to provide the teacher and the student with basic concepts. In other words, all of the words and phrases are considered important for complete understanding of the subject.

However, it is easy to find important words and phrases or any kind of information in the books.

The Allied Health Occupations Series

Title	Format	Title	Format
Human Anatomy	Text	Orthopaedic Physician's	
Basic Chemistry	Text/Workbook	Assistant Techniques	Text
	Lab Manual	Respiratory Therapist	
Organic Chemistry	Text/Workbook	Manual	Worktext
	Lab Manual	Basic Microbiology	Text
Clinical Chemistry	Labtext	Introduction to Diagnostic	
Medical Office Practice	Worktext	Microbiology	Text
Cytology	Worktext	Medical Radiographic	
Basic Medical Laboratory		Technology	Worktext
Subjects	Worktext	Medical Mathematics	Worktext
Health Careers & Medical		Patient Care Techniques	Text
Sciences	Text	Dental Assistant Techniques	Worktext
Basic Medical Terminology	Workbook, Audio	Medical Records Technology	Worktext
	Teach Manual	Management Procedures	Worktext

In the front of each book a Table of Contents gives a general overview of each chapter, section-by-section. In the back of each book is a comprehensive Index that details information by word, by phrase, or by concept. Other built-in informational and instructional aids include charts, tables, drawings, and photographs that supplement and augment the text. Review questions help students as well as teachers judge the level of learning each step of the way, and suggested projects encourage students to practice and perfect professional skills. Specialized glossaries have been included where these have been deemed helpful for students.

All of the resources in the Series are generally interrelated to provide ease of use. Students and teachers need not readjust to completely different formats as they move from one subject to another. However, information is presented in a variety of styles to provide a change of pace that helps maintain interest.

About This Book

The book *Management Procedures* has been prepared as a guide for students interested in starting out on careers in the health care fields. It has been written for the novice, the beginning student who has had no background or experience in management. It can serve as an introductory text for a management course and provides much information on management procedures that could appropriately be applied to any of the Allied Health Occupations. The authors have kept the content general in nature and have maintained a simple but practical approach which should appeal to most students.

Health care managers find career opportunities in many kinds of organizations. Hospitals, clinics, nursing homes, and home health agencies are among those whose increasing needs for management personnel make this an important area of study. Although the areas of responsibility may vary greatly among these organizations, most of them face the same kinds of basic problems. Such common problems often revolve around an attempt to reconcile the ideal management system with the hard facts and limited choices that confront the health care manager in everyday administration. *Management Procedures* was written especially to provide essential guidelines for a prospective manager. The book covers the problems of interpersonal relationships, communications, person-nel management, and work organization. It discusses motivation and the practical aspects of organizational planning. It explores problem solving techniques and the philosophical and ethical aspects of management. It considers the use of computers in a medical setting and provides an introduction to computer terminology.

The text was written by Robert F. Comte, M.T., who is Adjunct Professor of Continuing Education at Mercy College, Dobbs Ferry, New York, and by Leslie W. Lee, M. T. (ASCP), who is Assistant Director of Laboratories at Orange Memorial Hospital, Orlando, Florida, and Clinical Assistant Professor of Allied Health Science at Florida Technological University, Orlando, Florida. Both authors have had wide experience in teaching and working in the management field.

Reviewer for the book is Ruth Williams, M. T., who is Professor at the University of Florida, College of Health Related Professions, Department of Medical Technology, J. Hillis Miller Health Center, Gainesville, Florida. Professor Williams states in her review, "This book should be a welcome addition to the libraries of those institutions where courses in management are offered. It fills a special need for specific information for managers in health care. It is liberally illustrated, is easy to read, and provides the basic information for further study."

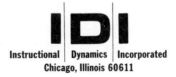

Instructional | Dynamics | Incorporated
Chicago, Illinois 60611

Philip Lewis, Ed.D.
President IDI

Linda J. Thomas
Editorial Director

Eleanor L. Bartha, Editor

Jane P. Barton, Associate Editor

Sophia A. Kaspar, Indexer

Contents

CHAPTER 1. **Our System of Health Care** 9

Hospitals and Their Employees, 12; Hospital Work as a Career, 14

CHAPTER 2. **What Is Management?** 16

Approaching Your Problems, 16; Attitudes and Habits, 18; Managing Your Time, 19; Your Resources, 21

CHAPTER 3. **Personnel Supervision: Hiring and Training** 24

How To Find Good Employees, 24; How to Train Employees, 28

CHAPTER 4. **Personnel Supervision: Interpersonal Relationships** 33

Characteristics of a Manager, 33; Characteristics of Employees, 34; Communications, 36; The Territorial Imperative, 41; Challenge to Authority, 43; Human Needs and Motivation, 45

CHAPTER 5. **Work Organization and Staffing** 52

Organizational Plan, 52; Job Descriptions, 55; Procedure Manuals, 56; Evaluations, 56

CHAPTER 6. **Computers in Medicine** 59

Patient Records, 59; How Does the Computer Do It?, 60; Hospital Applications, 63; Management Applications, 65; The Status-I Laboratory Based Computer System, 66

CHAPTER 7. **Physical Resources: Repair and Maintenance** 70

Arrangement of Space, 70; Inventory, 71; Care of Equipment, 71; Obsolescence and Deterioration, 75

CHAPTER 8. **Purchasing and Leasing** 79

Leasing, 79; How To Lease Equipment, 79; Cost Analysis, 82; Purchasing, 85; How To Prepare a Bid Request, 86; Glossary of Leasing Terms, 86

CHAPTER 9. **Finances** 90

How To Prepare a Budget, 90; How To Stay Within a Budget. 92

CHAPTER 10. **The Road To Success as a Manager** 95

Levels of Success, 95; Responsibilities, 98

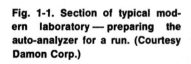

chapter 1

Our System of Health Care

In 1900, only 350,000 people were involved in health care in any way. For every doctor, there were only three medical workers to perform all of the supportive functions, and most of these persons were nurses.

By comparison, nearly 5 million persons now work in the health industry. Fewer than 1 in 10 of this army is a doctor of medicine. About 125 health occupations can be identified, and many persons work entirely within the "health community" at jobs that are not peculiarly medical.

Fantastic changes have occurred in the field of medicine during the past few decades. One could list dozens of innovations that have produced great changes in our general health, which were undiscovered two or three decades ago. Each important innovation has brought about changes that have demanded new products, new training, and additional personnel (Fig. 1-1). The discovery of the adrenal cortical substance ACTH, for example, made necessary the development of an entire field of pharmacology. New products were produced and marketed, new laboratory tests proved valuable, and new treatments were devised. For example, flame photometers for determining sodium and potassium levels in the blood and urine were

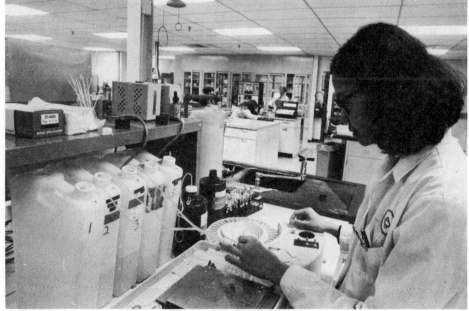

Fig. 1-1. Section of typical modern laboratory — preparing the auto-analyzer for a run. (Courtesy Damon Corp.)

developed. As a consequence today several large companies employ thousands of persons who produce, sell and service flame photometers. Furthermore, the use of intravenous solutions was revolutionized and many formulations of intravenous fluids were introduced for correcting fluid and electrolyte imbalance. These developments led to the development of still other new ideas with their own wide repercussions. Hospitals have become large, complex institutions, each employing hundreds of persons in all sorts of specialties. In addition, clinics, medical laboratories, health maintenance organizations, health insurance companies, and government agencies work together and among them employ millions of persons as part of the total health industry.

During the past decade the costs of medical care have risen rapidly. Much of this rise was caused by the increased complexity of medical equipment and methods. Part of it was necessary to bring the wages paid to medical workers up to a level reasonably close to those of workers in other fields. For many years, nurses and technicians were paid on an unrealistically low level. The great increase in demand for health care that came as a result of Medicare and health insurance made it necessary to train, employ, and hold more workers, and a salary adjustment was necessary. At the same time a rather high inflationary rate pushed all prices and wages upward.

Regardless of the reasons, medical costs became so high that the average family "could not afford to be sick," and major illness could wipe out a family's entire savings in a few days or weeks. Medical insurance rates had to be adjusted upward. When these rates are projected to cover the entire population for increased medical services that should be available, it is going to be necessary to find ways to get more medical care for the same amount of money. The ways in which this goal may be approached are really what we wish to consider in this book.

As health care organizations get larger, they tend to become bureaucratic. Persons who direct and organize work become interested in their own reputations and in the records of their own sections or departments. Often the larger goal of the organization as a whole is entirely forgotten. In this atmosphere, it is not surprising that sometimes persons at the bottom of the ladder lose direction and interest and are only concerned with whether a

task is in the job description and whether they are legally required to do it.

One fundamental fact about all health activities is that the patient (and indirectly the general public) is the only reason for their existence (Fig. 1-2). This may sound trite but it is too

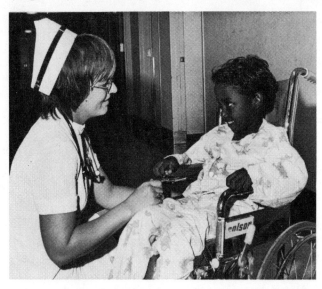

Fig. 1-2. Nurse with a patient.

often forgotten. Everyone involved in caring for the patient has his own particular duties to perform and his own standards of performance for measuring his effectiveness. These may occasionally militate against the well-being of the individual or the public in general. For example, a well-meaning secretary concerned with collections may be proud of having completed the necessary forms for every patient admitted during her shift. Her persistence in attaining her goal, however, may have left a patient so distressed with his economic plight that he was in no condition to accept the doctor's advice about relaxing and forgetting outside problems.

One would hope that the general objective, throughout, would be to enhance the efficiency of the system and that this would improve care. Ideally, decisions based upon such objectives would always be best for the patient, but any experienced administrator knows that sometimes solutions are not that simple. The good of the patient must always be the paramount concern.

Another concept that seems obvious is that doctors of medicine must have the final decision concerning patient treatment (Figs. 1-3, 1-4). This too may sound trite. In practice, such logic may lead to painful and difficult decisions since patient

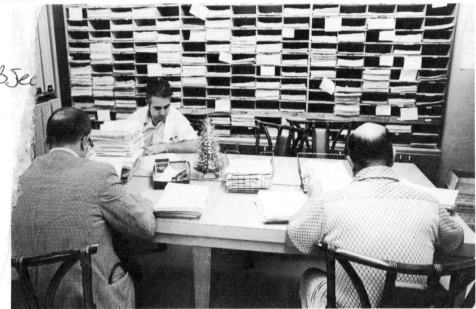

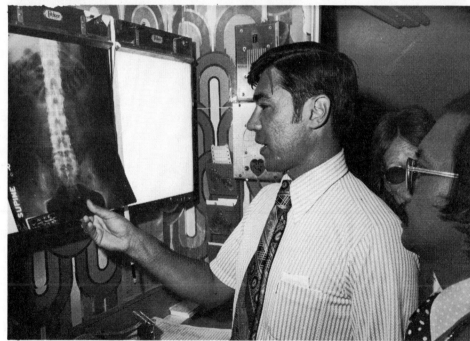

Fig. 1-4. Doctors checking x-ray view of spine.

treatment is closely tied to economic matters and organizational problems. Occasionally an administrator, a manager, or an employee interprets a policy decision in such a way that it interferes with the doctor's orders which were based on sound medical judgment. An example would be the adamant refusal of a technician to draw blood for a crossmatch and transfusion from a seriously wounded but unidentified patient. An error in identity could indeed lead to a transfusion accident and possible death with the concomitant possibility of a lawsuit, but without the transfusion the pa-

tient might die from loss of blood. The doctor must make the final decision.

The person at the head of the hospital is called the administrator or director. He may be a doctor of medicine or a person trained as an administrator. Whatever his background, the administrator must be in firm control of the administrative aspects of health care. He may occasionally have problems in reconciling his views with those of the physicians but these problems are his domain and, once resolved, he must have the management control to expedite his decisions.

Thus we have patient care (1) oriented to the patient's welfare, (2) directed by the physician, but (3) managed by whatever administrative person or team is delegated this responsibility. Ideally, there is no conflict inherent in this arrangement. Unfortunately, things are not always that simple and, as our system becomes more complex and specialized, "the forest may be completely obscured by the trees."

Central to a manager's creed is absolute integrity. The patient, the employer, and the employee must feel that he will be fair, impartial, and true to his principles; if they do not he will be unable to function effectively. This integrity must involve among other things a sense of loyalty, both to the organization and its administrative team and to the employees under the manager's control. A strong, stable organization cannot be built without it.

Modern health care institutions of all types and of all sizes need managers—informed, skilled, technically competent people—who have a liking for their job and empathy with patients and their fellow workers. This text is designed to give the student some guidance in the skills of management. Considerable space is devoted to interpersonal relationships and the ethical considerations that should determine their direction. It is our belief that the manager's concept of his job is the paramount influence that affects his performance.

Management means achieving the best possible performance with the resources at the manager's disposal. Goals are met by individuals. Unless the manager can bring together competent persons, train them, motivate them, and keep them functioning smoothly, the assigned task will suffer. Hence it is axiomatic that the manager must have a strong personal concern for the persons with whom he works. Sometimes other objectives must suffer to protect a qualified person or to keep a group from being sacrificed. As we shall see, wise choices are often hard to make when we weigh the ethical ideas such as those we have just considered against personnel needs.

It is often in the attempt to reconcile the ideals of management with the progress and growth of the institution that the manager faces his greatest problems.

Health care managers can be found in all types of organizations and specialties and the areas of responsibility may vary a great deal, but the basic problems, dilemmas, and frustrations often revolve around the same set of choices.

Since this text is addressed to the general subject of management, little space has been devoted to the details of operation. For the functional details of various hospital departments and their interrelationships, the student is referred to the fine texts on hospital organization and administration that are available.

Hospitals and Their Employees

Inasmuch as most medical workers will be employed in hospitals or will relate to hospitals in some way, a review of hospital organization is in order. There are, of course, many types of hospitals, both general and special, and they vary widely as to size, corporate set-up, and type of patient accepted for treatment.

Most patients are treated in general hospitals, which may be operated by non-profit corporations (the largest group); federal, state, and local governments; religious orders; charitable organizations; and physicians, either singly or in groups.

The administration usually rests with a hospital administrator or director who has earned at least a master's degree in either business or hospital administration. He has thorough knowledge of the functions of the various hospital departments, as well as the financial, legal, and managerial skills necessary for the direction of the hospital's affairs. He is answerable to a board of trustees, which sets general policy and develops the programs that are executed by the administrator and his staff.

Major Departments

Accounting. Like a family, the hospital operates on a budget, and it must live within its means. The trustees generally set certain goals and priorities and the administrator is responsible for collecting and spending funds in the best possible way to achieve those goals. The first priority must be the delivery of good quality health care to the patients. After that comes improvement of staffs, buying new equipment to keep up with new developments in the field, and providing for the physical growth of the hospital.

To help in the financial management of the hospital, a comptroller or treasurer keeps control of cash flow and of all the financial matters. The collection of patients' bills and the payment of bills for materials and supplies, as well as the payroll, generally are supervised by the comptroller. This function is carried out by the "accounts receivable" section of the department. Since most bills are paid by insurance companies or government agencies, the job is not simply one of accepting money in payment of bills. Charges from all the service departments are accumulated to make up the patient's bill. Charge tickets or vouchers for all of the services must be kept on file to prove why a charge was entered on the bill in case a question should arise. Completed bills are itemized and sent to the insurance company, to the individual patient, or to whatever agency is responsible for payment. The various companies and agencies that are responsible for the patient's bills may demand innumerable details of financial transactions and establish regulations that complicate the collection procedure considerably.

The "accounts payable" section is involved in calculating employees' work time, making adjustments for social security, income tax withholding, overtime, etc. Many records must be kept, and reports, surveys, and audits keep this section constantly busy. The processing of the hospital's bills for such items as drugs, food, supplies, and equipment is also assigned to the accounts payable section.

Personnel. In a large hospital, a personnel office recruits, screens, tests, and hires new employees. Here, employment records showing absences, illness, vacations, holidays, pay rates and raises, job performance records, and other details are maintained. This office also helps the administrator formulate personnel policy.

Purchasing. The purchasing department buys all supplies for the hospital. Thousands of items — from potatoes to penicillin and from beds and plumbing supplies to chemicals and medicine — flow through the purchasing department. In addition, the department arranges for the payment of all this material, as well as for utility bills, insurance contracts, leases, and service agreements. The process of selecting, buying, stocking, receiving, and issuing these supplies requires much space and many people. In these times of shortages, the problem of guaranteeing that no one will lack needed supplies becomes especially critical and difficult.

Maintenance and Housekeeping. The maintenance department, under the direction of the plant engineer, has the responsibility for the care, repair, and maintenance of the physical plant, including the buildings, equipment, and grounds. In a large hospital this can be a huge responsibility, with miles of hallways, hundreds of rooms, and millions of dollars worth of equipment. Nearly every trade — plumbers, painters, steam fitters, air conditioning engineers, gardeners, and electricians —is represented.

The housekeeping section, with a small army of maids, porters, and domestics, must keep all rooms and hallways swept, dusted, scrubbed, and neat. The collection of waste materials alone is an enormous job.

Pharmacy. The pharmacy issues prescription drugs and medications to virtually all patients. Seriously ill patients may have several medications each day, and many of these may be perishable, dangerous, or hard to obtain. A mistake in medication can be very damaging, or even fatal, to a patient. The pharmacy is among the hospital services that produce some of the revenue needed to offset hospital costs for which patients are not billed. A registered pharmacist is primarily responsible for the operation of this service.

X-ray and Radiology. This important service also produces revenue which helps with non-billed costs. In addition to taking and processing x-ray pictures, the department may perform fluoroscopies, cobalt or radium treatments, and conduct other types of examinations or treatments that employ radiation in some form. A physician who specializes in the practice of radiology administers the treatments and oversees the work of the technicians who take and process the x-rays.

Pathology Department. In its laboratories this department conducts thousands of tests on blood, tissues, and various body fluids. It performs complex analyses and examinations to help diagnose patients' conditions or control their illnesses. This is another revenue producing department that helps to pay the bills.

Respiratory Therapy. In recent years the respiratory therapy, or inhalation therapy, department has developed into a sizable operation that makes an important contribution to the care of patients. The administration of oxygen and various medications that can be inhaled is its principal function.

Dietary Service. The dietary department prepares meals for patients and employes and provides the special diets required by many patients. In many hospitals, this department may be "the biggest restaurant in town." The mechanics of preparing and serving appetizing, hot meals to patients in beds all around the building (or buildings) is a formidable task for the dietitian and her staff.

Nursing. All of these and other departments serve the patients by closely coordinating their activities with those of the nurses, who are ultimately responsible for patient care. The nursing service is the largest single group of employes. There will probably be one nurse, aide, or orderly for every patient in the hospital. These persons are most intimately involved with the patient and, indeed, provide for his every need while he is in the hospital. In addition to the floor nurses who give routine nursing care, there are many surgical nurses, coordinators, administrative aides, nurse educators, etc., who provide other service directly or indirectly to the patients. The registered nurse (R.N.) is the central person in the care of patients but there are many levels of specialties and of training. Licensed practical nurses (LPNs), nurse's aides, orderlies, and ward clerks are all part of the nursing team.

Emergency Service. Most hospitals provide emergency care for nonhospital patients through the emergency room. Doctors make fewer house calls and, in these days of mobility, many persons do not live in one community long enough to ac-

quire a "family" doctor to whom they can turn in case of need. When a person has difficulty finding a doctor for any reason, he is likely to come to the hospital seeking help. Since most hospitals will never refuse aid to anyone who is really sick or injured, many indigent persons who need help but are unable to pay their bills find their way to the hospital. Also, many patients are brought to the hospital emergency room by fire and police departments, or are sent there by welfare agencies, and even by their own physicians. Such public service has been thrust upon hospitals in many ways, and most have developed rather large facilities to provide emergency services.

Hospital Work as a Career

As we have seen in the foregoing section, the hospital is a complex, busy place with much challenge and responsibility. Many big jobs are accomplished by thousands of very dedicated people. If you would be a manager, the responsibilities are great and the work is demanding. The rewards in satisfaction and self-realization are generous. Financial rewards are not great but are usually adequate. If you would join the army of wonderful, valuable, dedicated—mostly fulfilled—persons in the hospital business, you will find many hands ready to help you along. But you must earn your own way.

Review Questions

1. How has health care changed in the past 25 years?

2. Name some factors that have caused the health care industry to increase in size.

3. What characteristics do you think a manager in the health care field should have?

4. Who is the most important person in a hospital? Why?

5. Who makes the final decision about patient treatment?

6. What is the head of the hospital called?

7. What is his function?

8. How do you define management?

What Is Management?

We commonly confuse such terms as direction, supervision, administration, and management. Many jobs may have elements of all of these but the words do not necessarily mean quite the same thing. At times it is hard to say which element predominates in a given job situation. Let us consider these similar but distinct functions.

A director directs the affairs of an organization by establishing goals and priorities that determine the direction the organization will take. The director might not directly supervise or manage in a technical sense since his role is primarily one of broad policy making.

An administrator administers or runs an organization within the framework of the various directives and policies given to him. Strictly speaking, he is not the person who establishes the larger goals but a "technician" who knows how to make the organization move efficiently to achieve its purpose.

A manager takes charge of the management or oversees the functioning of an activity to achieve a set goal or purpose. His strength is in his ability to use all of his resources to get things done properly.

A supervisor oversees the activities of others to get them to accomplish specific tasks or to perform scheduled activities most efficiently.

Many jobs that carry considerable responsibility have elements of all of these functions. Thus, the director may supervise the heads of departments or managers who will execute the directives he generates, and the supervisor may establish certain goals and priorities that could constitute direction. A manager will probably make little progress unless he is able to supervise the activities of persons under his control.

In reality, everyone who has responsibility for a section, an office, a laboratory, any activity—functions as a manager. He must make the best use of personnel, money, space, equipment, and other resources available to accomplish prescribed tasks in the best way possible. Management, then, is not a remote academic exercise but is the daily application of knowledge and good sense. It is our hope that the ideas we shall discuss may help you to organize your thinking and activities so you will manage your particular area of responsibility most effectively. We are not concerned here with establishment of broad policies in health care nor are we concerned with the mechanics of the administration of specific programs. We shall, however, consider in some detail the supervisory skills that may help to provide the manager with the means to achieve the desired results with the personnel at his disposal.

Approaching Your Problems

Good management involves orderly thought processes. Let us look in a general way at the sequence by which a manager may analyze his situation and set out to improve it.

On assuming his role the manager needs first to define exactly the task or function involved. This may be a very simple task, such as cleaning rooms (Fig. 2-1) or washing sheets (Fig. 2-2), or it may

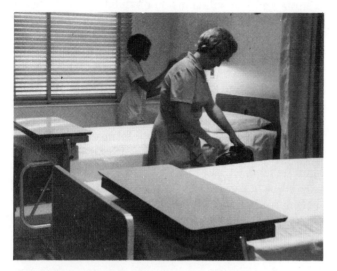

Fig. 2-1. Housekeeping crew preparing patient's room.

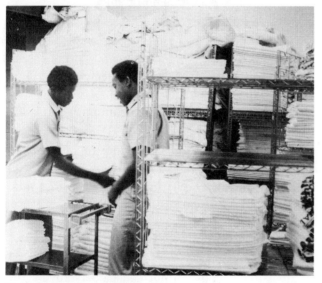

Fig. 2-2. Laundry dispensing linens.

be considerably more complex, such as the performance of all nursing duties in an intensive care unit. Even the simplest task needs defining. When completely defined, it, may be found to be less simple than was at first supposed. Do not try to spell out every activity at this stage of your thinking. In general terms you should ask yourself, "What are we instructed to do?" You will not be the first person in this situation to find that you are not quite clear about your assignment. If you cannot clearly define your task or responsibility, it

would be wise to discuss it with your superior until you have your objective clearly in mind.

Next, list those elements of the job that are important to satisfactory performance. If, for example, the task involves washing dishes, you might feel that (1) getting the dishes completely clean, (2) finishing them by a reasonable time, and (3) returning them to the serving line in neat, well arranged loads are the most important aspects of the job (Fig. 2-3). At this time it might also

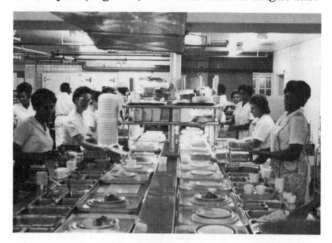

Fig. 2-3. Patients' trays being prepared on a moving belt.

be well to list actions and behavior that make the performance unacceptable, for example, (1) excessive breakage of dishes, (2) loud noise close to the dining room during meal time, (3) allowing the dishwasher to overflow so that waste water runs into grocery storage area.

Now look at the present performance and discover which of the desirable criteria are being neglected or left unsatisfied as well as the frequency with which unsatisfactory incidents continue to occur.

We have now clarified what we set out to do. We have established some criteria for good performance and recognized some areas of bad performance. With these as a guide, it is not difficult to measure present performance. Obviously, we will want to do better in most cases. In order to make our efforts most effective, some plan must be formulated to channel efforts and resources in such a way as to solve the most immediate problems and deficiencies.

Let us suppose that your most pressing problem is that water from your dishwashing room has three times run into the storage room and soaked into bags of flour and sugar, and the dietitian has promised to have your head, or words to that effect, if it happens again. At this point you establish an objective for yourself—namely, that the problem will be solved in such a way that any recurrence of this particular disaster will be prevented.

The first thing to do is to define or identify the problem concisely. This is another way of asking, "What really happened?" On examination you find that a dishwasher drain is stopped up with paper napkins, which causes water to back up. There is an overflow drain that should catch the waste water but it empties on the floor. If the washer is stopped in time, there will be no overflow but there are times when everyone leaves the room at once. Even when they are there, some workers do not know how to turn off the machine. Once the water starts across the floor, no one thinks to sweep it toward the drain or move the bags of flour and sugar off the floor.

Now put together a plan of action that is likely to accomplish the objective. First, itemize the contributing factors as follows:

1. Drain plugged by napkins.
2. Overflow not functional.
3. Personnel not present to stop machine.
4. No one knows how to stop machine.
5. No one sweeps water to drain.
6. No one moves the bags of flour and sugar.

Then list the steps to be taken to solve each deficiency:

1. Train all personnel to be sure no napkins stick to plates going to washer.
2. Have maintenance department reconnect the overflow pipe.
3. Establish a strict rule that the washer is never left unattended.
4. Train all personnel on steps needed to shut down the machine in an emergency.
5. Buy an extra broom for the dish room and make sure that everyone understands that it is imperative that it is used when the water is rising.
6. Suggest to the dietitian that the sugar and flour could be stored on a shelf above the flood area.
7. Ask the maintenance department to raise the door sill to the grocery storage area.
8. Take the dietitian to lunch soon and discuss your problem amicably.

9. Check every week on all steps that have been initiated to be sure no recurrence of the problem is possible.

Not all of the manager's problems will be this simple and the solutions so obvious. In most cases, any problem becomes simple when it is clearly stated, and the solution then becomes easier. Sometimes, however, you may not be able to decide whether the problem has been solved without some actual measurement or judgment being made. If this is the case, such criteria should be established in advance and a schedule decided upon for applying them and re-examining the problem.

In many instances, the logical steps to be taken can be chosen easily, but the problem is never solved because of failure to follow up on the initial action and, either the orders were never actually carried out, or they were misunderstood, or action was discontinued as soon as the problem seemed on its way to solution.

Attitudes and Habits

If we review the process we have just gone through, we will find that we have analyzed our operation, found the most immediate problem, and established its solution as an objective. Solving it involved the following steps:

1. Identifying and clearly defining the problem.
2. Examining the causes.
3. Choosing appropriate steps to offset these causes.
4. Reviewing the situation for possible additional solutions or relevant points.
5. Taking action.
6. Reviewing the results and following up on action.

Most likely you will not consciously follow this sort of procedure each time problems arise, but following a reasoned, logical process should become a habit. In learning to swim, ride a bicycle, or drive a car we practice certain responses until we are no longer aware of deciding what to do next. So it is with various skills in management. We do not usually decide, "Now I will think about this problem and solve it." We simply do it more or less reflexively.

There is another quite useful thought habit that a manager should make a part of his nature. This is the practice of insulating himself from excessive emotional involvement with a problem. We are all in the habit of seeing the acts of others only in the perspective of their effect on us. We may see another person's actions as personally offending us, and we almost unconsciously respond by defending our positions and possibly attacking the miscreant who offended us. Most of us have been trained, in the normal process of becoming adult, to contain our stronger emotions so we do not hit our opponent and usually do not even shout at him. But we resent him and in some way we let him know of our resentment. As a leader, we must train ourselves to react in a different way. Each time our authority is questioned, our project is damaged, or our position is compromised, we should consciously go through a thought process something like this:

1. Ask first why you are so upset. Be very honest with yourself. This will probably not be the same answer you would give if someone asked you because you do not want to sound petty.

2. Then ask why the rascal did this to you (or your project or plan). If you think it through, the chances are that he is responding to some fancied slight and if you were in his position, you would do the same thing.

3. Decide that the job at hand is too important to jeopardize by responding to the personal slight.

4. Look at the event only as it affects the job you are trying to do and react constructively to these problems.

5. If the offending person is one with whom you are often involved, talk it over with him and try to remove any hostility that may exist so that he will not continue to be a potential source of trouble.

Once it becomes a habit, you should find this process very rewarding. You will find your problems easier to solve; you will make new friends who, in turn, can help you, and you may establish your reputation as a good manager. Best of all, you can simply side-step the tensions and hostility that often make managing a painful experience. This process does presuppose a certain facility in handling people. Later on we will discuss ways that will help you develop your potential in personnel supervision.

Some wise man once remarked that before we attempt to manage others, we must first be masters of ourselves. Mastering ourselves is such a large order that hundreds of books, tracts, and sermons have been written about it. Rather than become philosophical, let us consider some very ordinary concerns that have to do with managing ourselves.

Managing Your Time

Most of us are plagued by the problem of never having enough time to do all the jobs that fall to our lot to complete. It may be that more jobs are assigned to us than we feel we can finish or we may project more for ourselves than we can ever accomplish in the allotted time. Experts tell us that our problem lies chiefly in organizing our work and our time. We can almost always explain to ourselves, and everyone who cares to listen, that we always wind up with the problems. Workers are not competent, we say, and no one really takes any responsibility. So, grumbling as we go, we put in a couple more hours' work and do the job ourselves and if we cannot manage to get it done, we may quite truthfully tell everyone "we just cannot do everything."

The truth probably is that we have failed to delegate as we should and have not made good use of our time. In most work groups, a careful examination will show that a few people do the largest part of the work and, for some reason, several people with good potential are simply not pulling their weight. In a later chapter we will talk about this problem but, for now, let us simply say that you are not very efficient if you are doing all the work and others are not working to their full capacity. Some managers even say: "Never do anything that you can get someone else to do." This may be overstated but the idea is sound.

So often we say: "The days just are not long enough. It is five o'clock and I am just now ready to start this project. I have had interruptions all day long." It seems that every time we start something there is a good reason we cannot proceed. With larger organizations, more directives, more meetings, and increased government control, there certainly are many interruptions and frustrations. If we take firm control of our own affairs, however, it is possible to organize our time so that we manage a good part of it. One way to start is to discipline ourselves to exact hours in the office or place of work. Next, we can analyze exactly what we do all day. You might be surprised if an efficiency expert told you exactly how

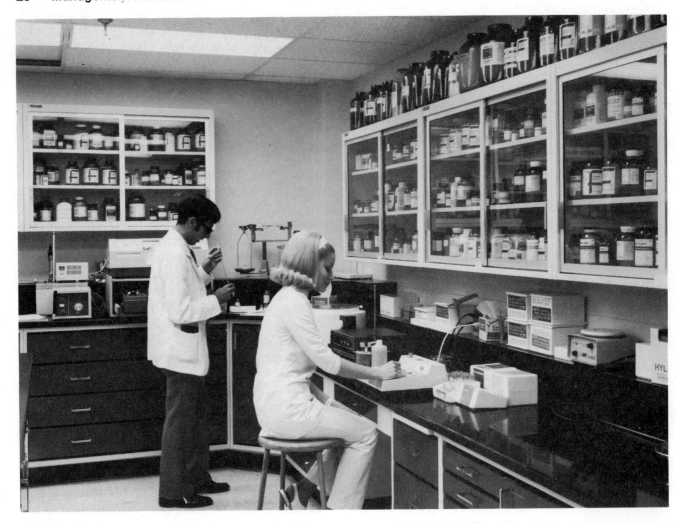

Fig. 2-4. Technicians in the laboratory. (Courtesy Clay Adams, Division of Becton, Dickinson and Co.)

you spend your time. Busy work and controllable interruptions probably account for a larger part of your time than you would admit. Jobs you could have assigned to someone else probably account for even more.

Following are a few practices that may prove helpful.

1. Schedule specific times for doing certain tasks. Sometime in the first part of the morning should be a good time to set aside for an uninterrupted planning period. It may be best to do this after hearing the problems of subordinates and receiving any directives from your supervisor. Your plan for the day does not have to look like a battle plan but it is well to set certain priorities and goals before the initiative is taken away from you by events and you are left indecisive. Quickly think through the most pressing situations, analyzing each

one and deciding what action must be taken to handle each (Fig. 2-4).

2. Set up certain office practices or job disciplines. Personal problems should not interrupt work unless they are serious enough to cause work problems. Then they should be resolved reasonably quickly or the problem person should be removed — temporarily perhaps — from the work situation.

3. Make certain that while conferences and telephone conversations are courteous and friendly, they are also brief and to the point so time is not wasted on trivia.

4. Do not accept a subordinate's responsibilities. Be helpful and patient but make it clear that the job remains his to do, not yours.

5. Do not put off unpleasant tasks. We all hate to face up to problems but often they are like dead fish or visiting relatives. After

three days they get worse. There is also a tendency for unsolved, thorny problems to accumulate if they are not dealt with promptly. Too many unsolved problems greatly weaken your control of the situation.

6. When several people need to be informed about various phases or parts of the same project, have a meeting and explain the whole process. You will avoid repeating information, everyone will understand the whole process, and you will also eliminate the possibility that you have given two people different impressions.

7. Set up an easy system for feed-back. You need to know that the plan you set up has been followed, that it is effective, and that it is not discontinued when your attention goes to other matters. If the feed-back system is made easy for the person who gives you information, he will be more likely to continue it. Acknowledge that you have received the information and comment on it so that he will know you are still interested in getting it.

8. Periodically review your day-to-day procedure to be sure you are discontinuing time-consuming and space-consuming projects when they have no further value. If you have been doing the same job for five years, you almost certainly have a wealth of anachronistic procedures that serve no purpose but to take up your time.

9. Delegate as much work and responsibility as you can. Others will be happier to have some responsibility and recognition. You will get the job done with less effort and the person to whom you give the job may have time to do it better than you would have.

10. Do not be afraid of new ideas. If they sound as if they could possibly work, thank the person who gave you the idea and give him the credit. You will grow in his esteem and the idea may make your operation look better. If some part of the idea does not seem workable, accept and give credit for the whole suggestion and then tactfully discuss the dubious parts.

11. Be generous with praise and stretch yourself to understand and appreciate everyone.

Your Resources

Earlier, we defined management as doing the best you can with the resources at hand. For most managers, these resources are rather similar in broad outline.

1. Your greatest asset is the people with whom you work. These may include only your immediate crew, team, or staff but may also include your supervisor and your colleagues.

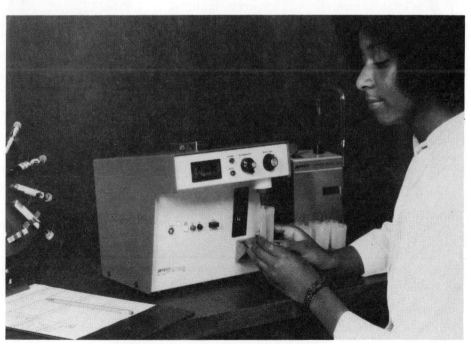

Fig. 2-5. Typical blood-cell counting equipment found in the laboratory. (Courtesy Royco Instruments, Inc.)

Remember that enough money will build buildings and buy equipment and supplies but only good management will develop an effective team.

2. Another large asset is your tools. This general term includes all the instruments, machines, and materials with which you work. In an office you will have typewriters, adding machines, files, forms, etc. Maybe you will have the dubious blessing of a computer. In the laboratory your tools may be spectrophotometers, cell counters, and all the instruments and materials needed for a medical laboratory (Fig. 2-5). A central services department will have autoclaves, sterilizers, instruments, and surgical supplies (Fig. 2-6). Whatever your tools, they are a resource and they must be cared for and managed.

3. Most sections or departments have a specific area in which they must function. Often the limitations of space are a serious impediment to effective performance.

4. Money is always involved in what you do. You may not personally handle any funds but they are still an important consideration in your planning—whether the money is coming or going.

5. Methods, work organization, and ideas are the principal ingredients of your management. It is by the organization and dispatch of your work, the innovations you make, and the general progress you generate that your success as a manager will be measured.

In subsequent chapters we will discuss the development of all those resources and the best ways to make the most of your people and tools.

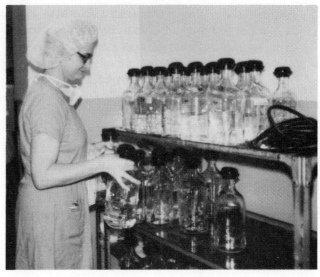

A. Preparing sterile solutions.

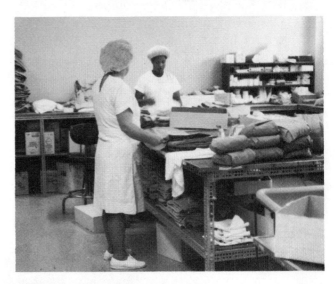

B. Preparing sterile surgical packs.

Fig. 2-6. Central services supplies.

Review Questions

1. Explain the difference between a director and a manager.

2. Think about a problem in a work situation with which you are familiar and apply the reasoning process presented in the chapter. Outline it completely on a separate sheet of paper.

3. List three thought habits that a manager should develop.

4. Prepare a list of general procedures and rules you would adopt if you were given a large office staff to manage.

5. How would you define management?

6. What general tools does a manager have to work with?

chapter 3

Personnel Supervision: Hiring and Training

The most important resource of any manager is his personnel. Compared to the total effort of his section, the work that the manager can do alone is insignificant. With a properly functioning team he not only can fulfill his mission, he can surpass it. The ability to supervise people is more important than any other single skill a manager may acquire.

Certain people seem to have an innate capacity to influence others, but the skill of getting people to function smoothly as a team can be acquired. There are many techniques that can be learned. As in any other field of knowledge, a certain amount of reading and study is required. You must be prepared to change your way of thinking and reacting. Self-discipline is important.

Individuals are remarkably similar in their wants and needs. In general terms, the bank executive responds in about the same way as the street cleaner when faced with the same situation. Persons who provide medical care are pretty much like everyone else, but some characteristics may be more common among hospital employees than they are in other occupations.

Not long ago most medical care was rendered by women whose sole motive was compassion for suffering people. One thinks of Florence Nightingale, the Angels of Mercy, and the many women volunteers who have nursed the sick and injured

solely because of love and a desire to help. This altruistic spirit is far from dead. Changes in our way of life have made it harder for individuals to devote their time and energies as freely as before but many nurses and other medical personnel are in their particular jobs largely because of the satisfaction they get from helping the helpless. We may be inclined to discount such motives but, as managers, we should appreciate this motivation and take care that it does not turn to cynicism through misunderstanding and frustration.

How To Find Good Employees

Among the persons who apply for jobs in medical surroundings, one may find a significant number of people who are somewhat neurotic. Possibly, persons who are unusually concerned with their health feel more secure close to medical care. At any rate, they seem attracted to hospitals and clinics. The number who are employed will depend upon the significance the employer judges this trait to have, the availability of other choices, and the effectiveness of the personnel department in screening applicants. The time lost by employees that is chargeable to illness is an important item in overall efficiency so it is wise to give this characteristic some consideration.

There are also, in the general population, a considerable number of persons who actually have chronic illness of some sort but appear to be healthy. A few diabetics, bleeders, epileptics, and others may find some security in being close to competent care. Because of the medical care frequently given as a fringe benefit in hospitals, they may be much closer to being able to pay their own way when they work in medical facilities than they would be elsewhere. Sometimes individuals who have had personal experience with illness identify more easily with patients and may therefore make good health care employees. However, one must always bear in mind the risk that some of these may lose considerable time from work and become a burden on the institution.

The medical field has a larger percentage of women than do most other occupations. We usually associate women with such roles as nursing, for example. Traditionally, a male nurse for female patients is considered entirely unacceptable and the same applies to many other hospital positions. Usually, women in work situations respond similarly to men but their motivation may be somewhat different because of family responsibilities and the conditioning of tradition.

Hospitals are complex social structures. A large hospital is like a small city with thousands of people using eating facilities, the laundry, utilities, nursing care, telephone systems, financial services, and even barber and beauty shops (Figs. 3-1, 3-2). People are busy 24 hours each day for seven days a week. Emergencies are constant and there is little respite between crises (Fig. 3-3). Human life is constantly in the balance; birth and death are always near. All levels of skills, from those of the most highly trained and skilled brain sur-

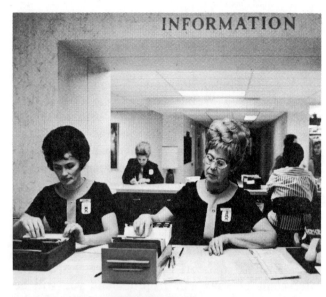

Fig. 3-2. Hospital information desk.

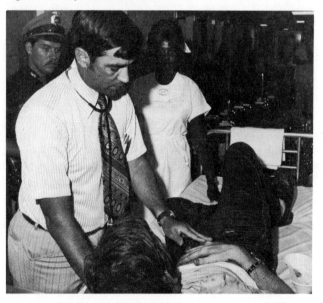

Fig. 3-3. Emergency room scene.

geon to those of the marginally employable person who scrubs the garbage chutes, are employed in hospitals. Within the same units, such as a surgical department, there may be persons of widely varying abilities and training.

This whole complex operation devoted to health care is nonetheless a business that must make charges, pay bills, and remain solvent like any other business. The efficiency with which managers discharge their duties and the ways in which their employees relate to the public determine, to a large extent, the reputation of the hospital and its success as a business. Success or failure eventually touches each employee in some way. The

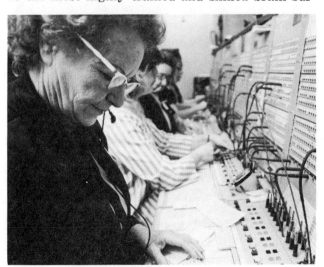

Fig. 3-1. Switchboard of a busy hospital.

efficiency of the hospital has a direct bearing on the amount that can be paid out in salaries, raises, and additional help. If the hospital is not financially healthy, new equipment and other improvements cannot be made. No one, of course, is very happy working for an institution with a poor reputation. The manager is ultimately the pivotal person on whom the success of the institution and the welfare of many persons depend. His ability to select the right persons for jobs is one of his important functions.

When one assumes a supervisory or management position, there will probably be a group of persons already assigned to the department. In other cases, the manager may need to build a team. Even if you start with a full crew, sooner or later some persons will drop out and you will be involved in personnel selection. Let us look at the process of finding and hiring desirable employees.

How To Conduct an Interview

In most institutions there will be a personnel office that refers applicants who are actively seeking employment. At times you may find yourself recruiting from any place you can. In any event, the employment interview should be carefully planned. Before the applicant arrives, be sure you have satisfied yourself about the job you are trying to fill. A job description should be prepared in advance, listing the specific duties of the proposed employee as well as the characteristics he should possess (Fig. 3-4).

The setting for the interview should be arranged so that there are no unnecessary interruptions and the applicant is comfortable and reasonably relaxed. Seating, lighting, and other details should convey a friendly but businesslike impression. Avoid making the applicant feel that he is on trial. Think about the information and impressions you wish to get from the interview. If it is available in advance, study the application form before the person arrives. Of course, you may be extremely busy and will have to do your best under the circumstances in the time that you have. In any case, here are general rules that may help.

Do not appear rushed. Try to put the applicant at ease by talking naturally about some common interest. Interspersing small talk about a place where you and the applicant have both been, a mutual friend, or a similar experience relaxes the prospect and he will be more natural. While dis-

Sample Job Description
Admitting Clerk

```
                            Code # 66454
                            Dept.: Patient Admitting
                            Salary Level  685-760/mo.
```

DUTIES:

1. Prepares patient's hospital chart prior to admission.

2. Assigns patient to specific hospital room.

3. Prepares addressograph plate showing complete and accurate patient identification information.

4. Discusses details of hospitalization with patient including costs, insurance and various procedures.

5. Takes patient and belongings to admitting nurse in reception area.

6. Accepts valuables from patients who wish vault storage of such items. Receipts all such transactions.

7. Performs any and all other duties, involved in the admission of patients, as may be assigned by the Director of Admissions.

Supervised by: Director of Admissions

Supervises: Admissions Typist and Porter when porter is assigned to her area.

Qualifications:

1. High School Graduate

2. Experience in Admitting Department

3. Experience with Addressograph card printer

4. Pleasing Personality

Affiliations: None

Fig. 3-4. Typical job description.

cussing places and people you both know you may be able to verify parts of his story, or discover omissions or exaggeration. At any rate, if you listen and watch you can find out how he handles himself in a meeting with a stranger. The quality of the language he uses, his sense of values, and his ability to express himself will all come out as you lead him into conversation and observe and listen. Be careful that you are not the one who does all the talking. Also remember to listen carefully and watch for hand motions, body language, nervousness, etc. We do not consciously judge all of these little signals that another person puts out but a composite judgment is formed, taking all of this subliminal information into account. All of the more-or-less subconscious judgments you make might be called intuition—but they should not be ignored when you reach a decision.

On the other hand, however, intuitive judgment may be faulty so we rely more heavily on those things we can actually perceive and evaluate. Look at the application form and study it for some of the following information:

1. Has the applicant written clearly and concisely? If his writing is sloppy, it may indi-

cate a generally careless attitude. If many questions are left unanswered he may be forgetful or evasive—or he may be expressing his unconcern for the whole process.

2. Can the dates of employment he lists be checked? Does the application provide a chronologic record for all of the time since he got out of school? If not, ask about it. He may be hiding a jail sentence, a psychiatric commitment, or a previous job record of which he is not proud. If there is no employment record and no explanation for long periods of unemployment, he may be inclined to loaf between jobs and to work only under duress. Look for many changes in jobs in a brief period of time. Job hopping may indicate a basically dissatisfied person or one who has undesirable characteristics you have failed to notice.

3. Can you picture him in this particular job? Be sure his training and experience indicate that he is capable of the duties you expect him to perform. On the other hand, over-qualification is about as bad as under-qualification. The highly trained or skilled person will very probably become bored with a simple, repetitive job or one that does not use all his abilities. It pays to have some mental picture of the type of person you have in mind. Without this you may be "shopping without a grocery list," and you may get someone who looks good but has little real value to you.

4. Do his degrees or certifications sound plausible and can you verify them? It is not uncommon for an applicant to present or imply credentials he does not have. On more than one occasion we have found that a job applicant has "borrowed" degrees and certification, and even a name, from a person who actually existed. Checking such credentials is difficult. Some knowledge of schools, professional requirements, and laws may help considerably in unmasking an imposter.

5. Are there some valid looking references you can check? Always check at least one of these. If the prospect is still employed in his previous job, it is reasonable for him to ask you not to call there for a reference. A reference at a fictitious address is cause

for concern. One bad reference out of several good ones does not necessarily provide a reason for rejection. After all, there are undesirable employers as well as employees. Sometimes an emotional firing and a bad reference may be the result of a genuine misunderstanding.

You should check to see if the person given as a reference is a close friend or relative of the applicant. A resident physician recently gave his mother (with a different last name) as his first reference. Also, the value of the reference will depend upon the credibility of the person who gives it. A peer of the prospect would be a better reference than a casual acquaintance. Beware of the sympathetic and non-specific reference. The unamplified statement that the applicant "is a fine Christian girl," or similar faint praise, is almost worthless.

6. Does the medical record contain many entries? Most application forms include some sort of medical history to be filled out by the applicant. If the medical history is lengthy or if there are several vague, undiagnosed symptoms, there is a good chance the applicant is either in poor health or somewhat neurotic. In either case he may be a poor risk as an employee. The application form should contain leading questions about mental and emotional problems and any history of alcoholism or drug dependency. A simple statement at the end of the application saying that falsification of the form is grounds for dismissal provides a simple means of discharging an employee with such a history if this becomes necessary and he avoided these questions or falsified the answers.

The advisability of employing applicants with epilepsy, diabetes, etc. might depend on several questions. Is the illness under medical control? What effect might the illness have on a patient, assuming the worst circumstances? Would time lost for illness be supportable? How obligated is the institution for continuing medical treatment?

7. Is there evidence of a previous criminal or emotional background? You may want to be public spirited and give a former prisoner

or an emotionally unstable person a chance. But the hospital, where each patient's welfare is at stake, should not serve as a proving ground for persons whose contribution to the efficient function of the institution might be questionable at the outset.

8. As a general rule, hiring relatives is frowned upon. It is not unusual for this sort of relationship to cause conflicts. The same applies to hiring close personal friends. In general, it is not advisable to hire members of the same family into the same work unit. This is especially true if one family member must supervise the other.

9. If other things are equal, hire people you instinctively like. The same characteristics that attract you will probably attract patients and other people. Such an empathy between your employees and those you deal with may help tip the balance in your favor when you need it most. Do have the good judgment, however, not to be swayed by a mini skirt or broad shoulders when the applicant has little ability.

10. In general, the person who must work for financial reasons is likely to be a more stable employee than is the person who is economically independent. Most of us have days when we would throw in the towel and go home if we could safely do so. The person who cannot easily do this is more likely to accept difficult situations as part of the job.

How To Train Employees

Once we have chosen the applicant we wish to hire, he should be told both the good and bad features of the job. If he takes the bad features in stride and the situation is better than he had imagined, he will be satisfied. If he feels you have hired him without telling him the bad features he may understandably be resentful. Most employees will rise to a challenge. Before they start to work, tell them the harder things you want them to do. They may accept your challenge as the norm and turn in a better work performance than you had expected. The people who will become strong employees may quickly accept a "missionary job" in which they have to put in extra time and effort

to solve difficult problems. The same person might not accept one which he felt did not challenge him.

Your institution will undoubtedly have some sort of standard hiring form that is easy to understand. If you are uncertain about how to complete this form and if it is your duty to fill it out, check with the director of personnel. Be quite sure that all details are correct and that you have been very specific about any special instructions. Pay differential for different shifts, dates of possible re-evaluation, etc. are very important to the employee.

Personnel Policies

The salary and the opportunities for advancement may not be within your authority to determine. Be as factual as possible about matters of personnel policy. If you really want an employee you may be tempted to be as optimistic as possible to entice him. This must be done with caution. If raises or advancement are implied because of the excellent performance you expect from him, he may resent not getting them if it turns out that his work is only acceptable. In this case you will have caused an acceptable employee to doubt your honesty or his own ability. Advancements and raises present very difficult dilemmas at times and the difficulty is compounded by half-promises.

Most organizations have a written policy that spells out work rules, vacation and holiday benefits, sick leave policy, and other regulations. These details should be given to the employee at the time of hiring if not before. If no policy exists, one should be prepared. The general outline of such a policy can be copied from that of a similar organization. All matters that are important to the employee should be stated as clearly as possible. Employee unhappiness is more often due to misunderstanding than to ungenerous treatment.

Orientation

A definite period should be scheduled for orientation. Unless this is done in an organized way, you may find that six months later the employee still does not know about things that affect his efficiency. In the orientation period, fellow workers, supervisors and people with whom he will come in contact should be introduced. The physical arrangement of the facility should be explained (Fig. 3-5). Questionable points concerning work rules and policies should be clarified. A brief his-

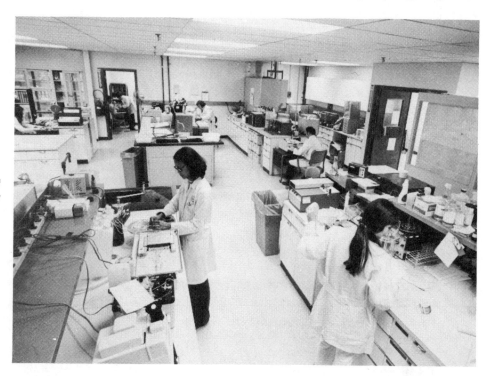

Fig. 3-5. Physical arrangement of a modern laboratory. (Courtesy Damon Corp.)

tory of the institution should be given. The orientation should help the new employee get his bearings in the work situation so he knows what he can do, to whom he can turn for help, and what he can expect to happen. The orientation session gives you the best chance to instill a sense of identification and pride in the job.

As a manager, you may not have the time to orient new employees. Instead of indefinitely postponing this important function, it would be better to delegate the duty to someone. Choose this person carefully for he will have much to do with determining the attitude of new employees (Fig. 3-6). When an older employee is given this

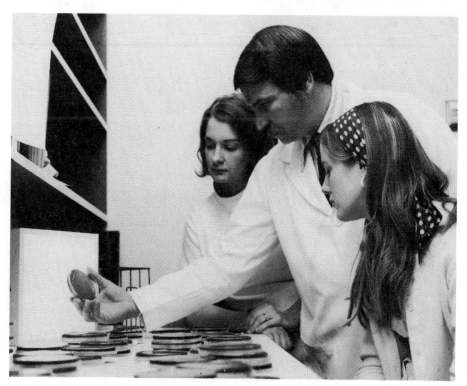

Fig. 3-6. Orientation of new employees—examination of culture in the bacteriology department. (Courtesy Damon Corp.)

task he may, in effect, sell himself on many of the good points of the organization as he presents them to the new person. By making the assignment you are showing your confidence in the person assigned and this may have beneficial effects. Some organizations assign different supervisors to orientation each time it is done.

To amplify the points suggested above, the following subjects might be covered in orientation.

1. Hours of work and appropriate comments about tardiness. Irregularity in reporting for work can seriously decrease an organization's efficiency.

2. Sick leave policy and the procedure to be followed if an absence is unavoidable.

3. Work responsibilities and work station assignment.

4. Any ground rules pertaining to overtime pay or work that may require extra effort.

5. Dates, time, and place for receiving his pay checks. Any ground rules about pay should be explained in detail.

6. The degree of accuracy and care expected of him.

7. Any rules pertaining to discipline or reprimands.

8. The employee's area of authority and responsibility. Misunderstanding arising from confused lines of authority can be very damaging to an organization.

9. The mechanism for settling problems and complaints. This should be clearly stated so that employee frustrations can be quickly sensed and dealt with.

10. Rules concerning care of property, including punishment for pilferage, negligent or willful damage of equipment, or defacing of work areas.

11. Opportunities for education, training and advancement. Some way should be found to prepare the employee for changes in his job or his schedule so he will be psychologically prepared to accept progress easily.

After the orientation period, or perhaps during it, a work assignment must be made (Fig. 3-7). The new employee must be challenged but not overwhelmed. The extent of his training and the degree of confidence and ability he has must be judged so that he can feel comfortable with the job. During the first few weeks, until you are sure you have judged well, pay close attention to his progress. Even the best managers can make mistakes that may be costly if they are not noticed and corrected.

It is a good policy to have a period of probation —usually about three months—during which you are judging the employee and he is judging the

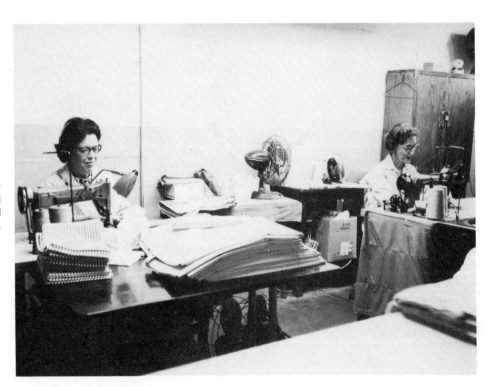

Fig. 3-7. An employee may be assigned to the laundry sewing room where linens are repaired and special items are made up.

organization. Frequent communication is necessary to help develop the worker to his highest level of efficiency and sense of satisfaction. A formal evaluation should be prepared and discussed with the employee at the end of his pro-

bation (Fig. 3-8). A report of this conference should be filed in the worker's personnel folder. Aside from the practical benefits of such a review, it is almost mandatory in many states because of provisions in unemployment insurance laws.

Employee Appraisal Form

DATE: _____

EMPLOYEE _____ DATE EMPLOYED _____ TIME ON PRESENT JOB _____

DEPARTMENT _____ PRESENT JOB _____ ABSENTEE RECORD _____

SCALE: (1) EXCEPTIONAL (2) VERY GOOD (3) GOOD (4) POOR (5) UNACCEPTABLE

CRITERIA	1	2	3	4	5	DOCUMENTATION (1,4,5)-COMMENTS
JOB PERFORMANCE						
1. Possession of necessary knowledge and skills.						
2. Application of principles and skills necessary for effective job performance.						
3. Quality of work: thoroughness, neatness, accuracy.						
4. Work efficiency; utilization of time.						
COMMUNICATION						
1. Relationship with co-workers.						
2. Relationship with superiors.						
3. Relationship with subordinates.						
4. Reporting of pertinent information.						
5. Attitude toward job - loyalty to hospital and lab.						
DEPENDABILITY						
1. Attendance						
2. Punctuality						
3. Flexibility						
4. Reliability - Completes assignments without being reminded.						
HOSPITAL STANDARDS						
1. Support of hospital policies regardless of personal feelings or opinions.						
2. Cooperation in maintaining safe, clean and pleasant hospital environment.						
3. Appearance and conformity to dress code.						
PERSONAL DEVELOPMENT						
1. Potential for growth.						
2. Interest and desire for growth.						
3. Participation in development and education programs.						

Employee Appraisal Form
PAGE 2

SUMMARY

1. Areas of strength and positive accomplishments:

2. Areas in which improvement or growth is needed:

3. Recommendations or comments:

Evaluated by _____

Position _____

Date _____

EMPLOYEE CONFERENCE

Date _____

Employee comments:

Employee's Signature

Evaluator's note on conference:

REVIEW

Reviewer _____

Position _____

Comments:

Signature _____

Date _____

Fig. 3-8. Employee appraisal form.

Review Questions

1. What characteristics do hospital personnel in general possess that may differ slightly from those of factory personnel?

2. Describe the preparations you would make for an interview with a potential employee. Use a separate sheet of paper.

3. With another student, set up an imaginary job and prepare a job description for it. Use a separate sheet of paper.

4. Make up or borrow an application form and fill it in completely. Use your own qualifications or make up the necessary information.

5. Act out an employment interview using the job description and application you have prepared. One student can play the part of the employer and another can take the place of the applicant.

6. What details should you spell out to a new employee?

7. Prepare a very simple personnel policy, making appropriate rules for the more important subjects that need to be covered. Use a separate sheet of paper.

8. (Alternate exercise in place of No. 7). Write a detailed sick leave policy as you think it should appear in a policy manual. Discuss it in class. Use a separate sheet of paper.

Personnel Supervision: Interpersonal Relations

All of us do some things well and, if we are honest with ourselves, we must admit there are other things that we do poorly. It is good for us to stop once in a while for a personal inventory. If we honestly judge our own abilities, it can help us in dealing with other people. Each person needs to make up his own inventory since he may have strengths that another person may never have considered. He also may have some failing, which never would be on the list of another person but which could be very damaging.

Characteristics of a Manager

After you have read the following characteristics that are desirable in a manager, take a few moments to make an inventory of your own qualities. Those listed here are a start but there are other traits, both good and bad, that you may wish to list.

Probably one of the most important characteristics of a manager is a liking for people. Interactions with people are like looking in a mirror. We get back an impression very much like the one we give in most cases. It is very hard to fool a person about your general feeling for him for very long. Your facial expression, tone of voice, eye movement, or a momentary lapse in speech will give you away. Charismatic people always like everyone. While it is true that some people naturally like everyone, it is also possible, by diligently studying the good, the interesting, the amusing, and the likable characteristics of those you meet, to cultivate a liking for nearly everyone.

A similar trait that seems to help is a natural optimism. The boss who is sure the whole organization is going "to smash" and that the bad guys will surely win has a hard time getting volunteers to leap on the wagon to take it where he is sure it is going. Optimism is actually deeply rooted in our own very personal sense of the order of things, which we call faith. We must feel that if we do what should be done things will come out right. Without some sort of faith in the rightness of our beliefs, there is nothing at all in our personality upon which we can build. The person who is basically cynical and pessimistic is sure to have a bad time as a leader.

Not only is a belief in "the rightness of things" necessary: one also has to believe in the rightness of the job he is setting out to do. It is very hard to get a person to do an outstanding job on a project that you do not believe should be done in the first place. It can be done, of course, but the task is much more difficult and the personal reward is hardly worth the effort.

As a part of his personality, it is necessary for a manager to have reasonably good self-esteem. This does not mean he must be an egotist but that he has confidence in himself and finds his efforts produce good results. It is difficult to be effective if you think you are unable to make good decisions or that your work is somehow not as good as that of the person you are directing.

If you are to build a successful group or organization you must want to do so. That is to say you must be ambitious. We often think of ambition as a deadly sin but a reasonable ambition to be recognized, to build, to work well is the very necessary starting point of all human endeavor.

In addition to the personality traits mentioned, there are many more tangible characteristics. For example, our manager needs self-discipline to force himself to do necessary things, even when they are unpleasant. Discharging a poor employee, for example, should be done as soon as it is obvious that it must be done.

Being a good listener is sometimes a frustrating task, but to do his job well the manager must be sure he has taken the pains to hear all relevant facts and points of view before making his decision.

Employees are very much affected by irritability, anger, and sullenness in their leaders. A pleasant, easy demeanor is necessary at all times and this is sometimes hard to achieve. Most managers have seen times when their failure to react in their habitual way has set up a chain of events that seems unbelievable.

Poise in the face of errors, disasters, and accidents is an important attribute. The manager who goes to pieces when things go wrong soon loses the confidence of employees who want to rely on him to lead them out of problems.

He must be accessible much of the time. If workers feel that there is no point in taking their problems to the boss because he cannot or will not talk to them, they will soon turn to others for help and advice as well as authority.

If he does not have a good memory for facts, people, events, etc., he needs to have an excellent set of records or a good secretary who acts as his memory. It is pointless to consult with someone who tomorrow has forgotten what happened today or what was supposed to be done.

Particularly, the manager must have a good sense of values and be able to make judgments where organizational goals and the well-being of his staff conflict. If goals which exceed the reasonable capabilities of the work force are set and relentlessly pursued, morale will eventually suffer. On the other hand, if the well-being of the work force is given such priority that work is slowed, the goals will be met in an indifferent manner and the morale most likely will not be good either. Ideally, of course, we would like to achieve the maximum operational effect with an enthusiastic and satisfied work force. There is, however, a level of productivity beyond which we pass only at the expense of excessive fatigue and disenchantment. The good manager senses this limitation and adjusts goals accordingly.

A composite picture of a manager, then, might be a person who likes and enjoys people and who has the self-discipline to plan and carry out his own affairs. He should be optimistic and believe in the rightness of the job he is doing and should believe that it can and will be done. He should believe in himself and his staff and be ambitious to succeed in his appointed task. He should be pleasant, poised and able to communicate easily with his staff by both talking and listening. He should remember what he sees, hears, and reads and be able to use all of this information in reaching sound judgments.

Characteristics of Employees

As has been suggested, persons who work in hospitals, clinics, and medically related organizations vary from those with very little skill to those with extensive highly specialized skills. Characterizing this heterogenous group by giving some common denominators is not possible. However, a few generalities might be made. A larger percentage of women work in the hospital field than work in industry, for example. Many career women are involved, but there are also a great many women who are the secondary bread-winner of the family. Because of their essential roles as mothers, many are forced to leave the hospital periodically and return later. The fact that qualified practitioners are constantly entering, leaving, and reentering the work force makes certain types of problems more common in the hospital than in industry.

In the first chapter we discussed the tremendous growth of medicine and the recent introduction of hundreds of new devices and techniques. Such specialties as respiratory therapy and renal dialysis employed only a handful of technicians 10 years ago; now the numbers employed increase every day. Training programs for some specialties are only now beginning to graduate appreciable numbers of technicians (Fig. 4-1). It is quite apparent that most of the workers in these fields will be younger than 30 years of age and in some

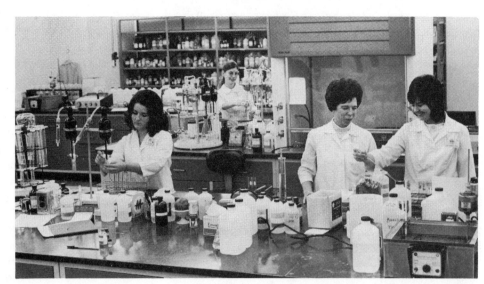

Fig. 4-1. Technician training program. (Courtesy Hycel, Inc.)

specialties, the average age is in the early 20s. Young people are often better prepared in many ways than are their fellow workers who are a generation older. They have a somewhat different view of life, however, and their motivation may be different from what has been accepted as standard in the past. In general, they are somewhat less competitive and more concerned about the qualities of life. Discipline, uniformity, and regularity may seem less important than freedom of choice,

ecological considerations, and work satisfaction. This is disturbing to some older managers. Certainly, it does not make management easier. This is not to say that the newer philosophy is not good or that older attitudes are necessarily better. There is little doubt, however, that there is a difference.

During the development of all of these new technologies the nature of education in the United States has also undergone a considerable change. The college graduate in the sciences today has a

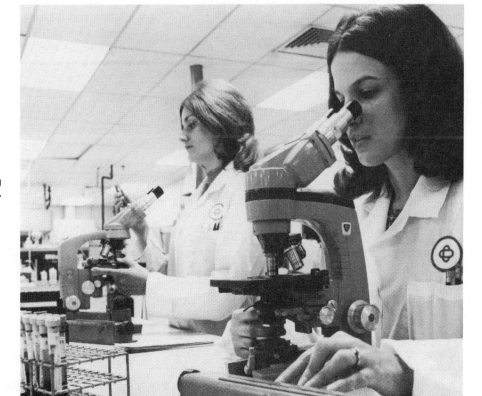

Fig. 4-2. Technicians performing manual blood counts. (Courtesy Damon Corp.)

much more detailed technical preparation than his predecessors had (Figs. 4-2, 4-3). It may be a problem for the older supervisor to cope with technically better prepared new recruits. If he attempts to overwhelm his charges with his superior knowledge, he may find himself on the defensive.

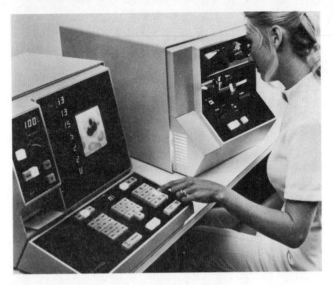

Fig. 4-3. Technician performing differential blood counts using a Larc Differential Counter. (Courtesy Corning Glass Works.)

Dealing With Different Motivations

How are we to deal with these different motivations? The woman who is the secondary breadwinner will most likely be concerned about the care of her family and will be less willing to work evenings or other irregular hours. Her prime motivation involves the well-being of husband and children and her ability to excel as a wife, mother, and homemaker. The supervisor who has to fill schedules is almost certain to be annoyed at the lack of flexibility of this sort of person, and for some situations this attitude is a real problem. At the same time, the supervisor should realize that he has built this limitation into the system when he hired this person. The secondary breadwinner may possibly be more permanent and better able to cope with repetitive or boring routines and, in many ways, may compensate for the lack of flexibility in scheduling. Recognize the prime motivations of an employee and use them rather than allow them to become a problem.

The callowness of the better prepared young employee may be an annoyance and his superior preparation may seem to be a threat to the older supervisor but a young, eager employee can really

be quite an asset. The supervisor should realize that experience and professional orientation give all the advantage needed to maintain control of the situation. The next step is to use his knowledge and to provide him with a means for moving up. The supervisor's reputation will be enhanced more by the leaders he has developed than by the talent he has discouraged.

The different values espoused by some young workers may be worth understanding. Admittedly, it is hard to schedule nights and week-ends using people who are more concerned with enjoyment of life than with the "rat-race." It is not unusual, however, to find that the "new breed," in addition to its other attitudes, has a very strong sense of concern and responsibility. Appealing to his altruism is likely to be more rewarding and more honest than are threats and coercion.

Communications

Whatever the group, the largest single problem in achieving a goal will probably be one of communication. It may seem amazing that in a society with a common language, a constant barrage of radio and television, the largest volume of newsprint in the world, and the largest telephone system that a problem of communication could exist. It is this very technologic complexity with all the advanced communications capabilities that complicates the problem. Words come to have different usages in different technologies and even where the words would seem to mean the same, there are slight differences in connotation. A directive that seems perfectly clear to an entire nursing staff may seem confusing to an administrator or an auditor. A very specific, informative laboratory methodology may be hopelessly confusing to a purchasing agent. Often these confusions are not a technical but rather a semantic problem.

Code Words

Still another problem arises from the fact that we are working with much more intricate methods, ideas, and situations than we were a generation ago. Explaining some of these takes many more words, and the actual time required to convey the idea becomes burdensome. For this reason we have come to employ code words to suggest ideas. For example, when an educator speaks of a "job ladder" he is referring to a basic idea in technical and vocational education having to do with preparing students to move from a lesser job to a better one by building on previous training. Those who have worked in vocational education have read and discussed the subject in detail and the two words "job ladder" bring to mind all of the common information associated with the subject. Each technology and discipline makes use of large numbers of such code words. When such expressions are used in conversation with a person of another technical background, the meaning may be totally lost. A few such code words mixed with commonly used words can provide a simple explanation for one person but are gibberish to another.

We are able to speak at the rate of about 125 words-per-minute. We can think at the rate of about 500 words. Hence we used code words, phrases, gestures, etc., as shorthand to speed up the transmittal of ideas. As we become accustomed to a code word, however, it no longer takes the thinking time of 50 words in our thought process. The code is one word (a discrete thought) which we accept at a rate of 500 per minute. If you listen for 10 minutes and hear 5000 words, it may take much longer to transmit the same ideas to another person who does not have the same word associations. More often than not we fail to realize that the words we use mean different things to others (or perhaps nothing at all).

As human knowledge multiplies and as we utilize ever more complicated devices and techniques, our communications become more involved. Bringing a new person into a discipline with which he is unfamiliar requires considerable communication. Fortunately, we are becoming more aware of the problem and our methods of relaying information are improving. As supervisors and managers we must learn what we can about all of the ways that we communicate and must continually be alert for ways to improve.

People living and working together develop many means of communication. Some are formal and obvious while others are so subtle that they almost escape notice or are so natural and inadvertent that we do not realize we are communicating. All of these are important to us. Let us think for a moment about all the ways we send messages to each other.

Means of Communication

When persons know each other well facial expressions are an economical and efficient means of communicating. Consider the wink, the raised eye-brow, the smile, a frown, a blank look, a skeptical look, or a cold, stern countenance. Can anyone doubt that a five-year old child gets the message that mother is angry without a word being spoken. An experienced speaker can read a quiet audience and tell how each person is receiving his message. A good supervisor can usually tell how his instructions or ideas are being accepted without a lot of conversation. He should be constantly alert for facial expressions as well as written and spoken messages. In fact, in small, close-working groups, much of the daily communication may be carried on without words.

In a similar way we communicate by body language. We consciously nod or shake our heads, point, shrug our shoulders, and make certain expressive gestures. These may be done wordlessly to economize speech or may be used to reinforce something we are saying. In either case they are very useful and should be used wherever they are appropriate.

Often we send unconscious messages by means of body language. We drum our fingers and reveal nervousness or impatience. We step close to a person to talk intimately or face him squarely when disagreeing. We lean forward to unconsciously express interest in a speaker. Sometimes we slump, expressing boredom. The person who carefully observes people will detect many subtle movements, changes of position, and postures that convey much information. Some of these may be very useful. We often sense these subtle messages subconsciously without being able to explain exactly what it was that conveyed the change of a listener's attitude or state of mind. We may tell ourselves that we have known instinctively. Careful use of body language can tell a person that you trust him, that you do not have the time to discuss a subject, or that you are annoyed or pleased. This means of communication can be economical and subtle.

Casual conversation is the most natural and often the most effective way to convey ideas. People vary a great deal in their ability to talk effectively. Practice helps but the sheer outpouring of words proves very little. Many very effective talkers use words very sparingly. Words are like tools that can be used to cut, chisel, or mold thoughts and ideas. In the hands of an artist they can produce a masterpiece, and a careless person can make a shambles of a simple idea. It has often been noted that a good vocabulary and success usually go hand in hand.

We can become more effective talkers with some effort. The advantages to be gained from improving our communications skills are well worth the work involved.

How To Overcome Bad Speaking Habits

There is much to learn and one can always improve. A few suggestions may give you a start and help to overcome some of the more obvious bad habits.

1. Speak distinctly in a voice loud enough to keep the attention of the listener but not so loud as to annoy him. Practice varying the pitch and inflection of your voice to emphasize points and provide variety. This makes listening much easier.

2. Use a few simple and expressive gestures but do not flap your hands or arms aimlessly. Gestures should be natural and comfortable to you.

3. Occasionally, write down what you have said —word for word. Go over it and eliminate the words that do not add anything to the meaning. Expressions like "I mean," "You know?," "I guess," etc., add nothing to your meaning and lengthen the time the listener must wait for you. Also analyze your sentences. Do you talk in complete sentences? Is your choice of words correct? Do you build from one thought to another or do you ramble? Do not impair your meaning by being apologetic or by unnecessary appeals to the sympathy of the listener.

4. Give the listener a chance. He likes to talk, too, and communication is a two-way activity. You can tell whether your ideas are getting across by getting feed-back from the listener.

5. Sound sincere and genuinely interested in what you are discussing. If you are caught up in your subject, you will come much closer to involving others.

6. Be economical in talking. Think before you speak and say just what you want to say. Do not get involved in details and side issues that do not reinforce the central idea you are trying to express. Use adjectives and adverbs only when they add to your message. The speakers who are most effective are very economical with words.

7. If you have the habit of interspersing "and uh" or "you know" every few words, break the habit. These are nervous habits that can be broken with self-discipline. Some people never end a sentence but splice everything together with "ands" and "buts." This habit also detracts from your effectiveness in speaking.

Properly used normal conversation with an individual or a small group is often the most effective and economical means of communication. Be certain you have said what you meant, however. A problem with this technique is that you get too relaxed and do not pay enough attention to whether everything was explained adequately. An advantage is that the listener can react by asking questions or offering suggestions or he can develop the conversation to see how you feel about what you are saying. This is, of course, the most natural and easiest way for most of us to communicate.

Group Discussions

If the group is larger or if the subject you wish to discuss is more involved, you may choose a more organized sort of verbal communication. Various types of structured meetings may be used. One should choose the format that accomplishes the job best and is the most natural.

If a new procedure is to be initiated, for example, it might be best to have a group discussion with all of those affected (Fig. 4-4). All pertinent details should be explained and a chance afforded for pertinent questions to be asked. The presentation should be thought out to be sure all details are presented clearly. Questions should be kept relevant but should not be discouraged. If you have failed to clarify some points, the questions are likely to help everyone. If there is a need to resolve problems, a conference or group discussion may be an excellent mode of communication. A plan or agenda for the meeting should be prepared. The moderator should guide the meeting but be careful not to inhibit discussion. The discussion must be tactfully kept to the subject under consideration and the tenor of discussion must be constructive. Organizing and moderating such a meeting requires some careful study and its effectiveness will depend in large measure on the skill with which it is organized.

Various types of structured group meetings can be set up for teaching. The manager's teaching abilities will have much to do with his success. He should seek any means available to improve them.

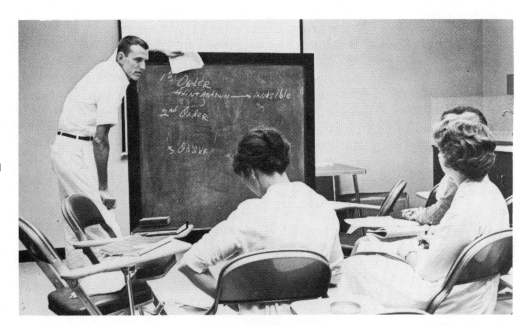

Fig. 4-4. Small instructional session.

Discussion with Individuals

The manager often spends considerable time in dialog with a single person (Fig. 4-5). The effectiveness of his communication in these sessions may be very important to his success as a manager. All of the various modes of communication that we have discussed may prove helpful. While it is quite important that these meetings be

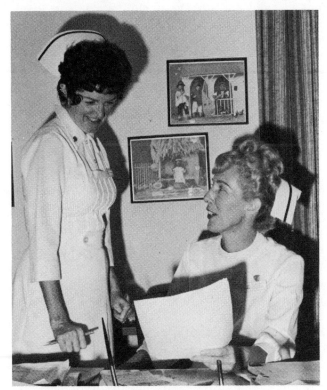

Fig. 4-5. Nursing director's individual consultation.

kept natural, effectiveness can be improved tremendously with study and self-discipline.

The important point in each contact is to accomplish the task or goal for which the meeting was planned: (1) An interview with a prospective employee is to learn enough about the person to be able to decide if you wish to hire him. You can also wish to convey to him certain things about the organization and its policies. (2) An evaluation conference is to let the employee know of his progress, encourage him, and suggest ways in which he can become more useful to the organization while improving himself. (3) A reprimand is to let an employee know that he has violated a rule and that you are officially taking note of it. You usually want to discourage him from repeating the offense; or, if you feel that he is beyond redemption, to establish documentation to support his eventual firing. (4) A planning or assignment meeting is to establish a course of action that the employee will follow. (5) A counseling session is designed to help the employee solve personal problems so that he will be of more value to the organization. (6) The complaint or grievance session is to solve problems that are causing difficulties.

All of this should be obvious, but we often forget the purpose of the meeting. In the interview, we spend much time talking about ourselves. In the grievance meeting we advertise all the things that annoy us. In the reprimand we justify ourselves, etc. Usually we set out to do the right thing but, while our words are saying one thing, our tone of voice, facial expressions, and body language are saying something else. Then we react to the other person when he chooses to believe the unspoken part of what we conveyed. Soon we are off the track and we never accomplish our goal. As we examine management practices, we shall look more closely at some of these problems.

The Written Message

At times written messages may be more desirable as a mode of communication. If we wish to document a rule, an event, or a situation we may write it for the reason of permanence. If we wish to get a message to a large group of people who cannot be easily assembled, it is more convenient to send or post a memorandum. If instructions or regulations are of the kind that must be consulted often, a written posted or filed memorandum should be used.

When a written message is prepared, the eventual purpose should be considered. For instance, regulations concerning penalties for tardiness and unexcused absences would be written in quite a different way from notices about the formation of an office bowling league, and both of these would differ from detailed technical instructions. This would appear to be obvious, yet many misunderstandings occur because the tenor, or tone, of the message was misunderstood. When we talk, the tone of voice, inflections, and choice of words tell our listener that we are asking politely, that we are explaining, that we are insisting, etc. When we write, we need to convey the same sort of message by the words, expressions, and general form of what we write.

Most of us have a great deal to read. It seems there is no end of letters, directives, instructions, inquiries, forms, and memoranda. If the general message is not clearly apparent rather quickly when we start to read, we lose interest and fail to read the material carefully. Any information we wish to pass on in a written message should be concise and clearly stated. The title or the first few words should be chosen to get the attention of the reader and tell him the nature of the information. It should also tell him whether and how it concerns him.

Often the writer of memoranda and instructions writes in terms of his own experience and needs. A directive written by a laboratory technician to nurses about the procedure to be followed for a test may explain exactly what he needs and what he will do with the information and materials requested and may even explain the significance of his request. It may, however, totally miss the details that the nurse may need to implement the directive. Consider the simple, easy instructions one might receive for a "serum rhubarb" clearance test:

"**We are now able to perform 'serum rhubarb' clearance tests which will be of great value in the diagnosis of 'China dropsy' syndrome.**

"1. Collect the total urine specimen each hour.

"2. Preserve with approximately 1 ml per liter of 0.1 NHCl.

"3. Send specimens to the laboratory after four hours.

"4. Urine and blood concentrations will be used to calculate clearance values."

The technician had written what seemed to him to be an informative instruction. He was irritated when a nurse called to ask where to get 0.1 NHCl and how much did she need. He explained that the containers were already prepared in the laboratory and the acid in each bag was close enough to the required amount. Some hours later he got another call asking how long they should continue taking hourly specimens. He was genuinely annoyed that she had not waited until morning when blood levels would be run. "Do we not always do blood chemistries such as this in the morning?" "Yes, but you did not say the urine test must be done at the same time as the blood," the nurse countered. "Well, how could the clearance test be of any value if the two cannot be compared? However, keep the urine and we will see what can be done." He went on to say that obviously the four hours the test had been under way was long enough.

Image his surprise when four hours later he was called in the dead of night and asked what to do with the urine for the "rhubarb" test. After waking up and calming down he called the nursing station to ask why the samples were so urgent at 2 A.M. "Well, the directions say send to the lab after four hours," was the reply. After a little profanity he went to put the urine samples away only to find one container with a copious amount of urine. He had failed to say that each hourly specimen was to be kept separate and the nurse had pooled them. He felt sure all nurses were supremely stupid and illiterate.

He had failed to say:

1. Where collection bottles are available.

2. What "approximately" means in this context.

3. When the test is to be done.

4. That urine samples should be collected each hour for four hours and preserved separately.

5. That after the last specimen was collected, all samples should be sent to the laboratory immediately.

Does this sound unlikely? Directions like this are written daily in hospitals, and confusion and errors are generated in large numbers as the readers fail to understand what the writer assumes that he wrote. In the foregoing example, the technician assumed that everyone knows that clearance tests are relating blood and urine levels at a given time. He assumed that everyone knows hourly specimens of urine in a case such as this are to be kept separate for a test on each. He assumed that everyone knows that most clinical chemistry tests are routinely started in the early morning. In short, he wrote the directive in the context of his own experience.

After any written communication is prepared, it should be read over carefully to be certain that all essential information is furnished. An example of a bad form is one that was recently received by one of the authors. It was to be filled out to verify the dates he would attend a meeting. All details were well arranged except that there was no possible way to determine to whom the form was to be returned or who could be contacted for further information.

A common error is setting a date and time for an important event only to find that the listed day of the week and day of the month do not correspond. For example, "All employees of this section must report to the personnel office on the 7th floor of the clinic building for reassignment before 9:00 A.M. on Monday, September 14th." On consulting the calendar, the employee finds that September 14th is Tuesday. Such mistakes are very easy to make and even proofreading often does not uncover them. It is wise to have a disinterested person read over written material to look for the obvious flaws that creep in.

If the housekeeping department is sending a notice to the nursing service, it is good to let a nurse read it first, to be sure that it is written in the terms nurses normally use. As in the case of the technician described above, we often talk and write in the context of our own thinking and experience.

Writing good, clear, understandable communications is a skill that requires study and practice. It is essential to good management in most circumstances. Take the time to learn to do it well.

When using a written message, take the time to be certain it is well done. Then review it to be sure it says exactly what you want it to say.

The Territorial Imperative

Some very interesting ideas about human behavior were suggested by a book written in 1966 by Robert Ardrey. In *The Territorial Imperative* Mr. Ardrey discusses animal behavior and suggests that there is a basic instinct that causes any animal to defend its geographic territory against any other member of his species. He presents many types of behavior that seem to be related to this instinct and draws many parallels with the behavior of people. The ideas are fascinating. Let us consider how the idea of territorial imperative may reflect in human behavior.

When a dog is in his own back yard he will defend the territory vigorously, even against a dog several times his size. On a strange street he will tuck in his tail and avoid all dogs, even those that are smaller than he is. We might say that humans have "backyards," not only in terms of real estate, but in terms of areas of supremacy of authority, knowledge, or interest. Whenever another person violates this psychological "backyard" there is at least an urge, an instinct perhaps, to defend it. If we watch individuals in their work environment, we are likely to see this idea in action quite often. If you have spent some time perfecting a system and feel that you know more about it than anyone in your work unit, you will almost certainly react when someone comes to your associates and starts telling them how "your" system should work.

This territorial reaction is not necessarily bad. In many ways it enables us to organize our activities better since the person who has been challenged will probably exert considerable effort to maintain his supremacy in such a situation. In the process he may exercise better control, do research on the subject for additional knowledge, and generally reinforce his position to the general advantage of the organization.

On the other hand, the manager who fails to take the territorial imperative of his people into account is likely to have considerable difficulty. Consider, for example, the new employee who has had good experience running a particular type of posting machine. If the person currently operating that machine has spent many months in that exact job, one needs to move very cautiously if the plan is to move the old employee to another job and put the new employee at the machine. Violating her territory, her area of knowledge and expertise, is an insult to her ego and one should not be surprised if she shows (or hides) some resentment. A possible approach would be to call in the present machine operator and compliment her on the way she has done her job (if that is appropriate). Then explain that she has the ability, knowledge, or skill to handle another area that is important. In other words, help her to define a new territory in which she can feel security and redefine her territorial imperative.

This sense of territory touches many situations. Our psychological "backyard" may include a geographic spot (an office, a desk, a town, etc.), persons (a special relationship with a superior), a piece of equipment, a process, an idea, or anything else in which we may feel some sense of proprietorship (Fig. 4-6). The good supervisor is sensitive

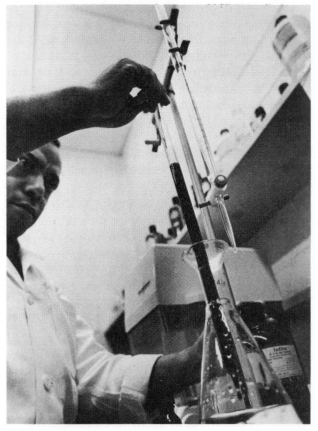

Fig. 4-6. Preparation of reagents requires precise measurement. (Courtesy Damon Corp.)

to the various territorial commitments of his personnel, and anticipates changes that may violate them and cause adverse effects. A genuine concern coupled with careful counseling can salvage many situations that could become very difficult.

This territorial sense is not always an individual phenomenon. Nationalism is a sort of territorial imperative and wars may start where two imperatives come into conflict. Thus the Jews, Christians, and Arabs all have a territorial identification with the city of Jerusalem and wars have gone on through the centuries because of it. In the same way, gangs, cliques, and other groups have the same sense of territoriality, whether it is the geographic area of a street gang or the ethical direction of a profession.

The "territorial imperative" can be used by a manager or it may work against him. If he is able to stimulate employees to feel that their organization and the attainment of its objectives is their own to defend and improve, he has a powerful tool working for him. If they feel no identity with it, they will perform their functions mechanically and a high level of useful activity will be harder to achieve.

If the group feels that it has a common bond in defending its entrenched positions and personal interests against changes made by the manager, he is indeed in trouble. Until he can convince all members of the group that improvements brought about by his direction are to their advantage he will have difficulty establishing his control. He will be unable to use their efforts effectively to improve the work situation. Stern discipline may, in the short run, get the job done but probably will not solve the underlying problem.

The Manager's "Territory"

The manager has his own territorial imperative, of course. It is natural for him to feel that his organization, his office and work area, his goals, and his ideas are his very own. A challenge to his authority, encroachment on his work space, or interference with his plans will annoy him. This is as it should be, for if he fails to defend these perquisites of his position he is likely to lose control and will not have the resources with which to work.

At the same time he may get into considerable difficulty if he is not flexible enough to change his position gracefully if the situation dictates such a change. He needs to choose his territory consciously to identify with the philosophy of his superiors and with the long-term goals rather than with his day-to-day decisions. This leaves him free to retreat gracefully from a bad decision and thank his critics for constructive help in solving his problems. His own ego will be satisfied that he has defended his position well and his critic becomes his ally who is also gratified by having defended his own position well. If the manager feels that a suggestion does not advance the organization's goals, he can discuss it constructively without fear of losing face. This, one might suppose, is the psychology behind the success of many men of high ideals and lofty goals. They are never in the position of defending a small decision or a petty circumstance.

Challenge to Authority

Various types of challenges often test the manager's authority, of course. Some are mere annoyances and some are serious. It is important that these be properly evaluated and dealt with. As we have just implied, the first consideration is whether the challenge is a threat to authority or is a responsible constructive criticism. Remember that the person who offers a valid suggestion has a position to maintain and, if he is summarily dismissed, he may become defensive and can pose an overt or covert challenge.

Rules for Establishing Authority

There are a few important rules in establishing and maintaining authority. One of the first is that poise must be maintained. In order to maintain poise it is important that you believe in your ability to handle situations. Most successful people decide that they will do everything they can to the best of their judgment and ability and will then relax and accept the ultimate outcome. If you can do this, much of the worry and uncertainty disappears and you can proceed calmly. If you have cut corners and then attempt to defend your errors, you will very likely "lose your cool" under challenge. This can be very damaging. People lose confidence in a leader who loses self-control.

Another rule is that authority must occasionally be asserted. This should be done by exhibiting positive leadership. Imposing negative rules may at times be necessary but establishing goals, setting work assignments, and demanding realistic productivity levels provide challenge and incentive without turning the worker off.

Fairness and impartiality are very important. The feeling among your employees that you have unfairly punished or rewarded an employee or have shown favoritism is very damaging. The feeling will persist that merit will not be properly rewarded and poor performance will not be punished so all incentive is lost.

As was mentioned earlier, the effective supervisor delegates as much as he can. This helps him get details out of the way so that he can concentrate on larger problems, but there is another benefit to be derived. If it is properly done, the person to whom work has been delegated will feel complimented and has, psychologically, accepted the supervisor as his boss.

Dealing with Challenges

The supervisor's authority may be challenged in a number of ways and it is well to recognize a few of these. One challenge is the employee who "butts in" and takes part in a conversation that does not involve him. He is the one who answers another employee's question before you have a chance to do so or gives advice before you can— or even after you have. He may be discouraged from the habit if you make it clear to him that you are talking to someone else and do not want to be interrupted. He may be miffed for the moment, but since his interrupting is primarily an attempt to get attention, you may enlist his good will by complimenting his work (if warranted) or by giving him constructive attention. This sort of challenge is annoying but not serious.

There is another sort of challenge which consists of an employee ignoring the supervisor's instructions. This can vary in severity from the employee who simply does not do things promptly or treats instructions casually to the person who very deliberately avoids doing what he has been instructed to do. The solution may depend upon the severity of the problem. If it appears that such a problem exists, one should first be quite certain that instructions are clear and that no other reasons exist for the work not being done. It is embarrassing to take drastic steps and then find that for some reason it was quite impossible for the employee to do the job. Often, employees are reluctant to explain problems to a new supervisor. The bearer of bad news is likely to be unpopular and they want no part of it.

After it is determined that instructions are clear and that the task can reasonably be done, the supervisor must hold the employee accountable for the job (Fig. 4-7). If it is still not done, counseling is in order. Often a calm, probing interview may uncover the cause of the worker's dissatisfaction and the problem can then be resolved. If this approach fails, discipline would seem to be indicated and if the problem is still unresolved, thought must be given to the advisability of transferring or dismissing the culprit.

Then there is the usurper who takes over the supervisor's role and assumes authority and responsibility. The situation may dictate the solution to this problem. If he's good at it and is not maliciously attacking the manager's authority, it may work to delegate some functions to him but clarify to him that you must have a chance to review his orders and amend them if necessary. With other types of usurpers, it may be possible to isolate the offender so that he is not able to interfere. If he is physically separated or given a task that is distinct from the tasks assigned to other employees, it may make it more difficult for him. As with the one who ignores instructions, the answer may lie in an in-depth interview in which his motivation is thoroughly explored. Often the problem is one of territorial imperative and a little careful work by the supervisor may reassure the employee and reestablish proper lines of authority without seriously damaging the employee's position.

One challenge to authority, which may become serious, is the bypassing of the supervisor. Employees may choose to go to the supervisor's boss and take things over his head. The best solution for this is for the offended supervisor to go directly to his boss and discuss the matter. If it is not resolved, this problem can become serious. Anyone who has supervisors reporting to him, should realize that lines of authority must be maintained. Responsibility and authority cannot be separated. If the person in charge does not relinquish authority the supervisor may find that his responsibilities have not been effectively delegated. If there is a difference of opinion between the supervisor and his boss that cannot be resolved, the supervisor might do well to consider his options and request redefinition of his duties or resign since his job will be a very difficult one.

The real challenge to a supervisor, however, is the "palace revolt," usually engineered by one or more organizers with the aid of rumors. This can be a devastating experience and it generally taxes all of the resources of a new supervisor. This state of affairs is usually the result of several administrative mistakes. Rumors are most effective in the absence of solid, factual information. If all of the facts about the employees' situation are discussed freely and often and if questions are answered immediately and frankly, rumor carriers have difficulty finding people to talk to. If there is general resentment, it is a pretty good indication that the territorial imperatives of many people have been violated without adequate steps having been taken to minimize damage that might occur to their prestige.

If things have gone this far, it is likely that some compromises will need to be made. The very first step is to reestablish communications. This may be painful and difficult but the supervisor must discuss matters until he feels that he understands exactly what is disturbing people. The real problem is usually not the first complaint voiced. The offense to one's dignity or to his ego may seem to the employee to be too trivial to discuss so another reason is found. Long discussion may be necessary and the supervisor must maintain his poise and flexibility. It is absolutely necessary that he feel and express his concern for the feelings of the aggrieved employees and that he reaches some accommodation with them on a reasonable solution to their problem. The real problem may be an insult to their dignity or their sense of territory and the solution may be a change of attitudes and intangible changes in emphasis. The agreement in words that is reached may be almost totally unrelated to the problem and may be meaningless. But it is still necessary so that the unmentionable in-

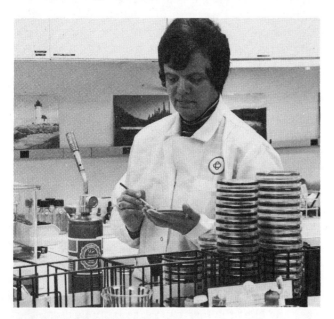

Fig. 4-7. Inoculation of culture medium requires care. (Courtesy Damon Corp.)

sults to integrity and territory do not become the issue and have to be embarrassingly dragged into the limelight. It is wise to emphasize that such issues as prestige are not minor and that you understand and sympathize when prestige is lost. Avoid discounting the expressed unrelated grievance, however.

Mending Fences

After the palace revolt is settled, it is a good idea to mend fences carefully. Communications must be maintained and the real problems attacked. Positive continuing measures must be decided on and diligently followed to be sure that the same situation does not develop again. If there are personalities involved that make it seem likely there will be a repetition, it is wise to transfer the offender, convert him to your point of view, or psychologically neutralize him so that he will not be a continuing threat to you.

It takes considerable time in a large organization for a new supervisor to gain effective control of the entire operation. In the next chapter we will discuss some of the steps necessary to analyze the problems and organize the resources. From the standpoint of interpersonal relations, however, the process may be slow and tedious. People must be studied so that the supervisor will understand personalities, interests, and reactions. Assignments must be made in ways that utilize strengths and avoid weakness. Often training, formal or otherwise, must take place to alter attitudes and habits. Mistakes are almost certain to occur and these may cost much time and effort. Almost as important, the work situation often changes rapidly and yesterday's goals and solutions lose relevance and new plans must be formulated. Particularly in the modern hospital, the supervisor's job is generally dynamic and a static operating plan is seldom achieved even though efficient procedures are eventually established.

The loyalty of employees is the greatest asset a manager can have. Management is not a popularity contest and one should not lose sight of this fact. Still, it is much easier to operate an efficient organization with the full cooperation and certain loyalty of one's workers. A few characteristics of human behavior should be kept in mind in working with people. Reasonable concern for these characteristics allows the manager to make his operation more successful, make employees more loyal and, at the same time, provide a work climate that is more enjoyable and productive.

Human Needs and Motivation

The psychologist Abraham Maslow has set forth certain needs that are shared by everyone. He rates these in order of their urgency and calls this classification "the hierarchy of needs." Various other authors have discussed his ideas and rearranged or restated them but his central thought is generally accepted and has had considerable influence on industrial psychology.

Before anything else, men need food and shelter. If they lack these basic needs, attaining them will be their first and most immediate consideration. Higher social needs such as status and security have little influence on the behavior of a hungry man.

After the basic physical requirements have been met, some measure of self-satisfaction is the next important need. The individual strives for some sense of his own worth and this need is quite fundamental. If he cannot achieve a good image, he will sometimes create a bad one in order to have a self-image that will at least provide some identity of self.

Once he has attained some measure of self-satisfaction, the individual will next strive for recognition by others. A great deal of our activity is, consciously or unconsciously, to achieve this recognition. Few mink coats would be sold if they were bought only for warmth.

All of us also have a desire to help others and, for some people at least, this seems to be a fairly basic need. In the medically related vocations, particularly, one would suppose this is quite an important drive which should not be dismissed lightly.

Having fulfilled the needs listed above, the individual begins to need to establish an identity and to be concerned with status. Social position and the accouterments of success now seem important to him. Titles, power, and a longer ranged security are now his needs.

Satisfying Employees' Needs

If we think about these needs in relation to the persons we supervise, we get some insight into the means for motivating individuals. We always move to satisfy a need, and the priority of these needs will be roughly in the progression in which we have discussed them. It is sometimes difficult to identify the motivation in these terms but the general concept is helpful.

For instance, the man with no money or resources will agree to almost anything to satisfy the basic needs of food and shelter. Once these needs have been satisfied, however, he may be entirely dissatisfied with the same job or conditions he had earlier accepted. This accounts for the large turnover in menial jobs where no self-satisfaction can be attained. Once the employee's basic physical needs are even temporarily satisfied he may find the elusive self-satisfaction in telling his supervisor to "stick it in his ear," if no other route to self-satisfaction presents itself.

Two points could be made here. In the first place, basic demands of the job should be made very clear to the employee when he has not yet started to work. He has more motivation then to agree to rules that he may dislike after he has been working for a while. Once rules are established and agreed to, there is a good chance to enforce them.

A second point is that some measure of self-satisfaction must be developed in the employee or he will be lost. If the supervisor acknowledges the efforts of the employee and, wherever possible, gives a compliment for work well done, the employee begins to satisfy this basic need and he will strive to do better. Even the very simple device of recognizing the employee as a person by a friendly "Good Morning," and a few comments about the weather will give him some self-satisfaction. Busy supervisors often feel that these niceties are of no consequence and are a waste of time. Actually, they are very helpful.

As soon as the employee has proved himself to his own satisfaction he may become bored unless he is accorded some recognition. Commenting to others in his presence about his good work often produces excellent results. This must, of course, be sincere and serious. If he feels that the comments are contrived or overdone, he may be negatively affected. Before the employee has achieved some self-satisfaction or conviction that he is doing well, he may not welcome too much recognition, since he may feel that he is the object of observation in an activity that he cannot perform. Very insecure people can be literally scared off a job by too early recognition.

Once the person has achieved a fair degree of recognition for his good work, he may possibly be used to teach others or to solve difficult situations. This step in motivation may be a difficult one. If the employee feels that he is being pushed into new duties for which he might be able to exact additional wages, he may seem perverse in his refusal to teach or help. Thus Mary P. may rebel at being designated as the instructor of new em-

ployees, but if a floundering new assistant asked for help she might spend extra hours showing her how the job should be done. If Allan K. is given the task of rooting out the cause of serious malfunction of equipment, he may try to side-step the job. If his supervisor confides his problem and deep concern and asks his help, he may immediately turn his full attention to eliminating the problem. Again, the approach must be entirely sincere.

The supervisor who is convinced that he really does not need his staff's help is quite likely to have a serious problem. Insincerity in personnel dealings stands out like a wooden nickel. It is, in fact, an insult to imply that you really do not need someone's help but order him to do a task to save you work or embarrassment. An honest straightforward request for personal help—help to solve an organizational problem or help for a person in need—is one of the most effective motivators for the employee whose more basic needs have been met. Many nurses and technicians, particularly, are real heroes for the time and effort they spend beyond the call of duty to help seriously ill patients. A serious plea for help for a sick patient is a high compliment to an employee and is usually taken as such.

An employee who has satisfied these basic needs, now requires, and has generally earned, some sort of identity. If he has not moved into some official position, such as supervisor, team leader, head nurse, etc., he may establish an unofficial identity as the best typist, most considerate nurse, etc., and be generally accepted this way by his peers. Every attempt should be made to work this person into the organizational structure for he will have considerable influence. If he is alienated, this influence can seriously undermine a supervisor or at least be an implied threat to the leader's territorial imperative and authority.

Identification with Group

A common problem is that of having an employee who has a strong territorial identity connected with a basic skill but has no sense of identification with the department or the hospital. This can create a serious situation and the supervisor should take steps to broaden the "expert" and provide him with a greater awareness of larger problems and responsibilities. Soreheaded specialists can be a menace to all concerned. Occasionally, all good supervisory efforts come to naught and the decision has to be made to lose a valuable employee in order to salvage morale or authority. If badly handled, this sort of situation can be damaging, whatever direction one takes. Early sincere and intelligent effort is indicated.

Assuming that the employee has moved successfully to fulfill all of his basic needs for identity to this point, his next need will be for status. This can be satisfied by salary or position. Considerable authority and responsibility may provide the needed status. Many leaders in the health field work under adverse conditions for relatively low salaries because of the status attached to the responsibilities they carry. Often they could go to easier jobs for more pay but find great satisfaction in status.

Curiously, money itself is not terribly important in any of these needs except as it is involved in the most basic ones. If the person cannot fulfill his physical needs on his salary it is desperately important, of course. More often it is a token of recognition relative to another person; or it is needed for a mother to help a child with something she wants the child to have; or it is needed to get a bigger car or house to establish status. This perspective makes it easier to help an employee meet his needs in the event that, as a supervisor, you can do little to change his salary. Satisfying the basic needs we have considered can be done in various ways. Largely in the gratification of these needs, individuals are motivated to do a better job. Since people always move to fulfill a need, we should never, as supervisors, discourage a need or want in an employee but rather should help him set up the criteria for meeting his need. All human progress is a story of people satisfying needs of some sort and the needs are, more often than not, more psychological than material.

Why People Work

People work for various reasons and it helps to identify the motive and classify the reason. The wife of a dentist who has grown children does not seek work for the same reasons that the young man with small children seeks it.

If we eliminate the basic need for money for food and shelter, the next most common reason for people working is their need for security. This may be security from dependency on someone else. It may be the security of financial independence for the older person with adequate but meager resources. Sometimes it is the security of working with familiar people in familiar surroundings at something the person can do well.

The housewife who stays at home alone a great deal may work for the attention and companionship she gets at work. Some people work for the satisfaction of accomplishment. The old carpenter who is financially independent may work for the sheer joy he gets from building beautiful cabinets and counters. Still others crave responsibility and are happy when they can be responsible for seeing that things are done. Some people need the approval they get for doing work well. For some people, work is an ethic and it is their serious responsibility to work even if it accomplishes nothing. Often people are much more easily motivated if we realize why they are here in the first place. A small raise in pay to the older dentist's wife is probably a poor motivation. Attention or approval might be very effective.

Almost all employees enjoy challenge, and boredom is deadly. We often err on the side of not giving people enough problems, for in problems there is challenge and in meeting challenge there is satisfaction.

Learn how to Listen

Much of the understanding of people that we must have in order to act wisely can be obtained by listening and watching. Most of us are so busy justifying ourselves that we fail to listen. Listening patiently and attentively is one of the better things you can do for someone. Talking to a sympathetic listener has a cathartic effect on the person who is talking and can convey much information to the listener.

Most of us fail to hear much of what we are told. Our attention span is short. We are busy thinking about what we are going to say next. We are distracted by mannerisms. We are not interested or we fail to "hear" the gestures, facial expressions, body language, etc. Often the real message is buried under various disclaimers. We treat the fulfillment of basic human needs, such as self-satisfaction, as suspect and probably not entirely honest. Even seasoned supervisors fail to realize the urgency of a very basic need, buried under double-talk about other people and other problems. Complaints are seldom about the basic need-fulfillment frustration that is the real problem. They will more likely be about some situation that makes the complainer look noble.

The wise counselor, however, treats the symptom reported by the complainer as the major cause officially while working out the solution to the bigger problem. Rejecting the non-problem may alienate the employee completely for it implies that he is not being honest with you.

Often employees come to a supervisor to discuss personal problems because they need an outside person to talk to and because they respect his judgment. They may also feel that the boss will understand their job failings if he knows about their personal problems. This sort of counseling can get out of hand rather easily unless a few basic rules are followed. The supervisor can be of help if he acts as a sympathetic listener. Rejecting the troubled employee outright can alienate him completely. On the other hand, becoming involved with the employee's problem can lead to totally unworkable relationships. Persistent problems of an emotional nature should be handled by an expert counselor, such as a psychologist, minister, or marriage counselor, and the supervisor fulfills his duty by advising the employee to seek such help and by helping make the arrangements where appropriate. Deciding just how far to go in counseling can be a problem with experienced supervisors since no two situations are exactly the same. Out of sympathy, one is inclined to allow infractions of rules. This is a dangerous practice that may later come back to haunt you.

Under no circumstances should the supervisor become involved with an employee socially or financially. Flirtations, lending money (other than very small amounts), or attempting to advise on emotional problems can all lead to disaster and, at best, may tend to interfere with the normal supervisor/employee relationship.

Winning the support and loyalty of the employee depends upon helping him to fulfill some of his basic needs. Giving him the job, if you have handled it well, should already have helped to satisfy a basic need and you have some advantage already. When criticism is made, it should be done as privately as the situation allows and it should be put in such a way that he will be able to see how improving his performance will be an advantage to him. That is to say, criticism should be constructive and made in such a way that it will build efficiency and morale.

Showing an interest in and an appreciation for the employee helps cement good relations. Questions about family, compliments about clothes, diet, hair, a new house or car pay big dividends if they reflect a sincere interest. We all like to think others notice the things that are important to us. Very few people would diet if they did not think the difference would be noticed by anyone.

Enthusiasm is contagious. If you show interest and enthusiasm for your work and for the people around you it will almost immediately reflect in the way people work and interrelate. We do not usually realize how much the moods and attitudes of the supervisor carry through the organization. The reactions of others generally mirror our own actions. Like looking in a mirror, when you smile at people they generally smile back and when you cuss, they cuss. When it is the boss, this effect is magnified. If he laughs often the unit is generally happy. When he fusses, the whole place has problems. Remembering this and using it to his advantage helps the supervisor control the tone of his organization without much effort.

It goes without saying that absolute fairness is essential to good morale. Once fair decisions are reached, discipline or reward must be equally firm and evenhanded. Favoritism must be avoided.

Supervisor Is Responsible

In the face of criticism from outside the unit the supervisor must be prepared to accept blame for his unit and take internal steps to rectify the situation later. You are responsible for the function of your unit. Do not under any circumstances, tell outsiders that Joe did it. You can correct Joe later. You will go up in his esteem if you take the lumps for the error, even if you pass them on later. If no error was made and your employees were blameless, go out of your way to brag about the fact that they do their job well and do not let them take unwarranted criticism. Just as they owe you some loyalty, you also owe them the same sort of loyalty. They will respect you more if you take their part when they are in the right.

When openings occur, look around and see if one of your own people wants the job and is capable of handling it. We often make the mistake of underestimating people's ability. Given proper motivation and training, it is surprising what reasonably capable people can do. You already know a great deal about your own people from working with them. A new person may present you with problems you do not already have and may be no more capable than someone you can immediately use. Promoting from the ranks improves morale and allows mobility for the employee without losing him to another organization. Training may be necessary but training usually has a double value because the instructor learns and organizes as he teaches and he may learn more than the person being instructed.

In general, we could summarize most of the foregoing by saying that effective supervision depends upon convincing the employee of the congruity of his needs and the needs of the organization. This is to say if he fulfills his role, the hospital (or other unit) will prosper and his needs will be gratified. Having convinced your employee of this, it is your duty to see that it is true.

Review Questions

1. Make up an inventory of your own managerial strengths and weaknesses.

2. How do you propose to try to correct your weaknesses?

3. Why should a manager be an optimist?

4. List as many of the ways in which you communicate as you can.

5. What are code words?

6. With another student perform the following exercise:
   (a) Student #1 explains what he thinks "Territorial Imperative" means. Allow about two minutes.
   (b) Student #2 explains the modes of the communication that were used by Student #1. One minute. should suffice.
   (c) Student #1 lists the ways Student #2 could improve his presentation.
   (d) Student #2 explains what "Territorial Imperative" means to him, profiting by the discussion in (b) and (c).

7. Write a memorandum, giving instructions about time, place, and preparation for the class you are now in.

8. What steps can you take to safeguard your authority as a manager?

9. What is the generally accepted hierarchy of human needs?

10. Should you try to persuade an employee's wife not to leave him?

chapter

5

Work Organization and Staffing

The chances are good that you will move into an organization that is already set up and you may not have much to do with initial planning and staffing. These are continuing functions, however. Over a period of time in most medical facilities, many changes occur that will alter the need for people or possibly even the basic objectives of the unit you supervise. Even if no obvious changes occur, it is a good idea to do a major review of the organization and staffing patterns at least once a year. The Joint Commission on Accreditation of Hospitals now checks such details every time it inspects a hospital and strongly recommends the annual update.

Supervisors often feel that organizational plans and job descriptions are nonessential bureaucratic devices. Actually, the organizational plan should be carefully thought out and should reflect the basic planning of the director or manager of the organization. Too often, organizations grow and change with little conscious attention being paid to the details of assignment of responsibility and authority. Job assignments, similarly, change with little serious thought given them, and impossible work situations develop before the supervisor realizes his dilemma. Effective planning is essential to good management.

Organizational Plan

Your organizational plan is a detailed diagram showing all of your people and their functions. From this it should be apparent who is responsible for each facet of the operation and to whom he is responsible. Often the lines of authority and responsibility are not clear. Preparing a diagram may demonstrate this to you. Perhaps someone has responsibility for functions but lacks the authority to execute them. It is not unusual to find that some employees either have no official supervision or are supervised by two people. While such arrangements could conceivably work for a while, the chances are good that they will eventually lead to disaster. Good management requires that each person be responsible and accountable to some supervisor. He should know who his supervisor is and should understand fully the nature and extent of his responsibility. Many misunderstandings arise between managers and supervisors and between supervisors and other personnel because someone does not understand the extent and limitation of his authority and responsibility.

The organizational plans of the clinical laboratory (Fig. 5-1) show how interrelationships can be depicted. Lines of authority follow lines from the top of the organization chart down through each echelon of authority. Chaos may occur when these lines of authority are violated. Work must be assigned by a supervisor only to the people whom he directly supervises and problems should always be brought to the immediate supervisor. Thus, if the laboratory director (see Fig. 5-1) starts to arrange the work schedule of the laboratory aide in routine hematology, problems will probably arise. If the technician in the automated methods section of chemistry takes his disagree-

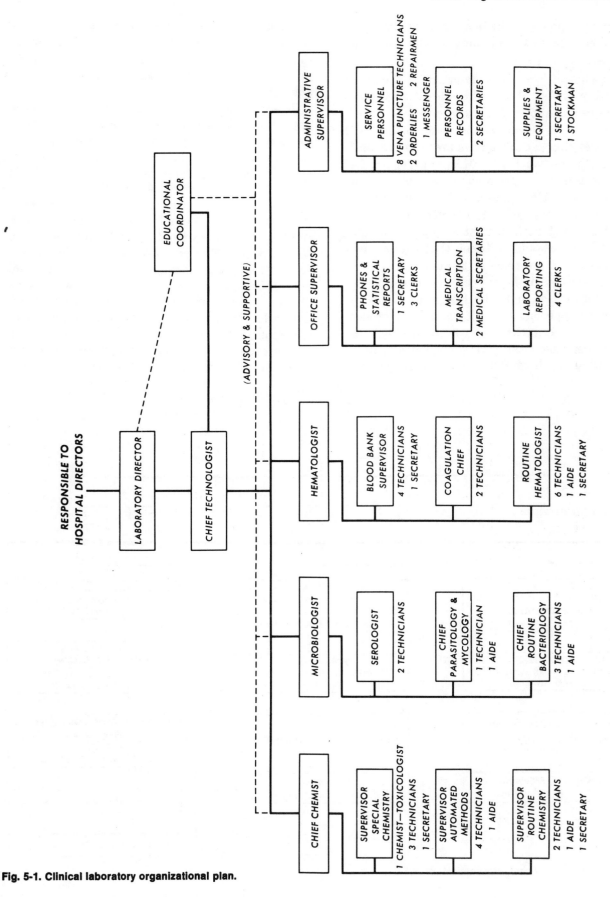

Fig. 5-1. Clinical laboratory organizational plan.

ment about supplies to the hospital director, problems are certain to arise among all the personnel concerned.

In the clinical laboratory depicted by the chart relationships might be further defined by additional diagrams showing the organization of various sections. Fig. 5-2 shows the section supervised by the chief chemist and shows areas of responsibility and lines of authority. Most supervisors feel that all persons below them should be able to come to them with problems and also feel they have authority to skip an echelon to correct an employee under them. Such actions must be kept to the minimum and care should be taken that the immediate supervisor is informed of the unusual actions. If an employee feels he is free to ignore his immediate supervisor and take his problems to his supervisor's superior, authority is quickly eroded. By the same token, the boss who passes over his crew chief's head risks giving conflicting orders and creating much confusion. Obviously, conflict-

ing orders force personnel to make decisions for which they are not in any way prepared, and if they cannot make the decision, or make an improper one, the whole operation may come to a standstill.

There is a definite limit to the number of people one person can supervise properly. Some authorities say four or five employees is the maximum. Certainly, one should not attempt to supervise people without a reasonable understanding of their problems and resources. Attempting the personal supervision of too large a group of people leaves the supervisor vulnerable since he may find himself finally responsible for work that he understands poorly. The people supervised are likely to feel that they lack adequate support and the whole enterprise may suffer. A wiser course would be to divide the group into teams, each of which can be handled by the person who has the most knowledge and experience.

The organizational plan should give a general outline of the organization and should show lines

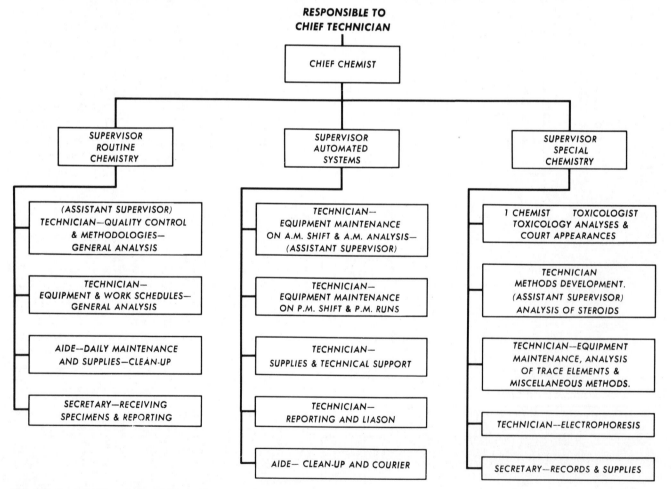

Fig. 5-2. Organization of chemistry section.

of authority and responsibility. It should show the relative position and function of each member of the group without ambiguity.

Job Descriptions

Each of the positions identified on the organizational plan must be described in detail by a job description. The title of the position should be reasonably accurate and descriptive. The duties of the person occupying the position should be listed completely but in general terms. Since methods and working arrangements change from time to time, the description should allow for performing the basic duties in any of several ways. An enabling phrase should be included to allow use of the employee in situations that are not listed. For example, the last duty may read: "Performs any and all other tasks involved in the posting of patient accounts." A general catch-all listing of this sort provides for utilization of the person in the solution of general problems in his area even though the particular problem was never anticipated when the job was assigned. Care should be taken, however, to list the employee's regular activities as completely as possible. If duties or responsibilities are shared with another person, this fact should be made clear (Fig. 5-3). If certain

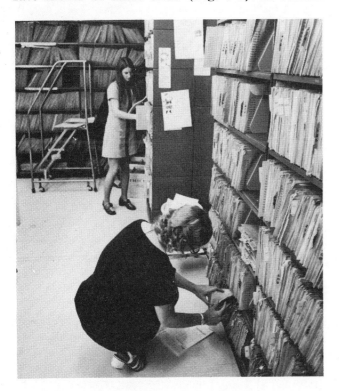

Fig. 5-3. Patients' records in medical records department.

functions are performed under the immediate supervision of someone else or independently, the fact should be noted.

The person to whom the worker is responsible should be indicated, as well as those whom he may supervise. The names of people are never used but rather the title. For example, the job description for the assistant comptroller might list:

"Responsible to: Comptroller"

"Supervises: All employees in Accounts Payable Section"

Qualifications of the person who could fill the job are listed. There is a tendency to list the qualifications of the person who holds the job. We should be more concerned with what the job actually requires. If an honest description is used it may even become apparent that the person in the job is under-qualified or over-qualified. Also, the honest listing of requirements for the job will help you when you have to fill the position with someone new. The listing of qualifications may include educational background, experience, skills, certifications or personal traits. Remember that accreditation rules or legal requirements may define some of these factors. You may wish to add other details to the job description, such as salary range, memberships and affiliations appropriate to the job.

A book is available which can be of considerable help. This is the "Dictionary of Occupational Titles," a publication of the U.S. Labor Department, available from the U.S. Government Printing Office. Descriptions borrowed from another source (such as this book) should be used as guides and should not necessarily be used verbatim. Often the job you are describing does not exactly correspond with the one in the book and there is no reason that it should.

It may be hard to decide just how specific you want the description to be. If the exact duties are listed in detail, you may describe a job that has grown up around the individual who is in the position. If you replace that individual you might never find another person who has this peculiar combination of talents and you might, in fact, not want the next person to concern himself with all these things. You might choose to say: "May also perform . . . . if qualified to do so" or "Performs other details of patient billing as may be assigned." If some care is not exercised, a separate description may be written for each person in the group, based on his particular duties and capabilities. Be sure to describe the job, not the person.

At the present time it may be necessary to code the job with a computer number that will identify various characteristics of the position. The ground rules of the coding pattern will be given by the programmer. For example, the first two digits may identify the department; the third, the specialty; and the last two, the level of skill.

Procedure Manuals

Even though you may feel that the work performed by your section is simple and easily understood, it probably lacks definition to a new employee. On close examination you may find that many aspects of the job are not really clear to you or to the older employees. Details should be spelled out in a procedure manual. This could conceivably (but not likely) consist of a page or so or it might be a small book. It should be long enough to give reasonably detailed instructions for all of the tasks routinely performed but concise enough to be easily read and understood.

The procedure manual should start by defining the function of your section in simple terms. It should then list all of the activities of the section and explain in detail exactly how each is performed. If appropriate, it should give criteria for judging if procedures have been successfully completed and should tell the reader where to receive help if it is needed. Much of the time spent in teaching new employees the details of their jobs could be eliminated by the use of properly prepared procedure books. If you were to investigate all of the errors and incidents of your sections you might be surprised to find that all of the people involved did not understand the details of procedure in the same way. The procedure book is simply an aid to better communication.

Evaluations

You should have some means of periodically evaluating the function of your unit. Many devices have been used to help you know if you are succeeding in your task. Some of these may be appropriate to your situation and others may not. You should establish the systems that would seem to tell you what you need to know.

Incident reports are designed to give various people the chance to report faulty service or a breakdown in normal routines. A periodic review of these gives a picture of what has gone wrong. An incident report form is shown in Fig. 5-4.

INCIDENT REPORT

"An incident is any happening which is not consistent with the routine operation of the hospital or the routine care of a particular patient. It may be an accident or a situation which might result in an accident."

PERSON INVOLVED

(LAST NAME) (FIRST NAME) (MIDDLE INITIAL)

MR. ☐ MRS. ☐ CHILD ☐ MALE ☐ FEMALE ☐ AGE

PATIENT ☐
ROOM NO. | STATE CAUSE FOR HOSPITALIZATION
PATIENT'S CONDITION BEFORE INCIDENT
NORMAL ☐ SENILE ☐ DISORIENTED ☐ SEDATED ☐ OTHER
WERE BED RAILS PRESENT YES ☐ NO ☐ UP ☐ DOWN ☐ ORDERED ☐ | WAS HEIGHT OF BED ADJUSTABLE YES ☐ NO ☐ UP ☐ DOWN ☐

EMPLOYEE ☐
DEPARTMENT | JOB TITLE

VISITOR ☐
HOME ADDRESS | HOME PHONE

OTHER ☐
OCCUPATION | REASON FOR PRESENCE AT THE HOSPITAL

EXACT LOCATION OF INCIDENT | DATE OF INCIDENT | TIME OF INCIDENT ☐ A.M. ☐ P.M.

PROPERTY INVOLVED ☐ EQUIPMENT INVOLVED ☐ DESCRIBE

DESCRIBE EXACTLY WHAT HAPPENED; WHY IT HAPPENED; WHAT CAUSES WERE. IF AN INJURY, STATE PART OF BODY INJURED. IF PROPERTY OR EQUIPMENT DAMAGED, DESCRIBE DAMAGE.

DATE OF REPORT | TITLE AND SIGNATURE OF PERSON PREPARING REPORT

NAME, ADDRESS AND PHONE NO. OF WITNESS(ES)

WAS PERSON INVOLVED SEEN BY A PHYSICIAN YES ☐ NO ☐ | TIME SEEN ☐ A.M. ☐ P.M. | WHERE

PHYSICIAN'S NAME | WAS PERSON INVOLVED REFERRED TO PVT. PHYSICIAN YES ☐ NO ☐

STATEMENT OF PHYSICIAN:

DATE OF REPORT | TITLE AND SIGNATURE OF PHYSICIAN

ADDITIONAL COMMENTS:

SIGNATURE OF CHARGE NURSE

Fig. 5-4. Incident report form.

Self-study evaluations are designed to allow everyone involved in your operation to review his own work and that of the section. Every facet of the operation is considered in detail to uncover strengths and weaknesses.

Statistical reports and financial reports are needed to tell whether the volume of work handled is as high as it should be.

Financial audits are very often necessary for offices involved in handling money. These examinations require accounting of all funds and a review of procedures.

Quality control systems are generally statistical systems set up to show errors in the quality of work performed. In laboratories they are essential for constantly monitoring the accuracy of laboratory tests. The Central Service department might use quality control to check the purity of distilled water or the sterility of surgical instruments.

Personnel evaluations tell the individual employee about his own performance and these should be done at least once each year. Care should be taken to discuss with the employee his strengths and weaknesses. His complaints, suggestions, and aspirations should be recorded. When this process is completed with each employee, the supervisor should consider the entire group and judge if he is making progress as a supervisor in improving the performance, the state of training, and the satisfaction of his group.

Forms, structure and organization vary from place to place. There is no magic combination and, like mankind in general, most of our organizations are imperfect since they are the product of imperfect people. As time goes along, more and more of medicine is controlled and standardized. Even though we may regret regimentation, we should not regard all organization and standardization as evils. Many of the forms, procedures and checks are means to our performing more adequately and productively. In this chapter we have looked at some of the dozens of forms that are rather fundamental to the successful operation of hospital departments. Many of these are required by law, registration, licensure, accreditation or custom and they have already defined many of our management functions.

We should look at these devices as tools to help us and not as the product of unbridled bureaucracy. Wherever it is your prerogative to review and evaluate the organization of your work, the forms you use, and the evaluative devices available, you should think carefully and select those that give the information needed with the least work. Organization is a means—not an end.

Review Questions

1. What purpose does an organizational plan serve?

2. Write a job description for the person who would clean up your classroom, listing the duties, qualifications, etc. as you suppose they should be.

3. How many people, like the cleaning person you have just described, do you think a supervisor could manage?

4. Name some ways the function of the housekeeping team might be evaluated.

5. What value does a personnel evaluation have?

6. How would you suggest quality control be maintained in the formula kitchen where normal babies' formula is prepared?

Computers in Medicine

With the phenomenal growth of health care facilities has come the need to process large quantities of information quickly and accurately. The population in the United States has grown from about 130 million in 1940 to more than 200 million in 1970. People use hospitals and medical facilities much oftener now than was formerly the case. In hospitals and other health facilities, much more information is generated on each patient. The number of individual bits of information acquired and stored has become astronomic. Consider the details of an average trip to the hospital.

Patient Records

When John Doe is admitted for chest pains he will probably stay for six or seven days. On admission, his name, date of birth, age, sex, marital status, address, Social Security number, insurance policy number and carrier, his employer, and name of closest relative must be recorded immediately. Usually, somewhat more information is taken. He is assigned an identification number, and his doctor's name and his room assignment are recorded. Details of diet, medication, laboratory tests and x-ray treatments, temperature and blood pressure are recorded several times each day (Fig. 6-1, 6-2).

Entries are made in his record by doctors, nurses, therapists, and technicians. He may have from 15 to 50 laboratory tests alone, (Fig. 6-3) and the entries of medications given may total several dozen during his stay. Each item of his treatment and care causes a charge to be initiated. These charges must be accumulated and posted to his account. They will then be forwarded to an insurance company or to Mr. Doe himself, and the collection file may become large.

During his stay, many different medications, special diets, linens, instruments and tools for his care must be provided, and the inventory, ordering, receiving, preparation, dispensing, and maintenance of these must be recorded. A small army of medically oriented employees, numbering about three per hospital patient, takes care of Mr. Doe, and their work time must be recorded and their pesonnel and pay records must be maintained. If Mr. Doe's hospital chart and files and his prorated share of the hospital's paperwork were put into one large box it is doubtful that he could carry them away from the hospital, even in the best of health.

As diagnosis and treatment become more rapid and effective, they also become more complicated and immediate. Also Mr. Doe has come to expect his care, meals, tests, treatment and bill to be quickly and efficiently prepared and available instantly. It is the way we have come to expect "instant" society to function. Like airlines, supermarkets, motel chains, and government agencies, hospitals have found that data handling has become their largest headache. Scheduling, the retrieval of information, billing, etc. have become so overwhelming that automation—largely in the form of computers—has become necessary.

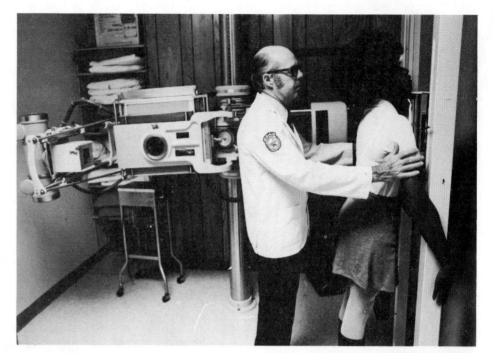

Fig. 6-1. Positioning of patient for chest x-ray.

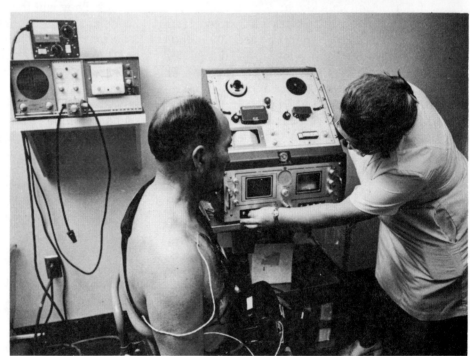

Fig. 6-2. Testing heart functions.

The problems involved in matching the capabilities of computers to the needs of hospitals has not been a painless process by any means. At the present time many hospitals do not use computers in any way and many others have only begun to use them for patient billing or other business records. In the next few years hospitals and other medical facilities will certainly become more and more computerized (Fig. 6-4). The present student of health management in nearly every field of medical care will need to know something about the unique capabilities and limitations of the computer.

How Does the Computer Do It?

The computer really is not a specific piece of equipment that solves all sorts of problems, as we are inclined to think. Actually, it is a group of in-

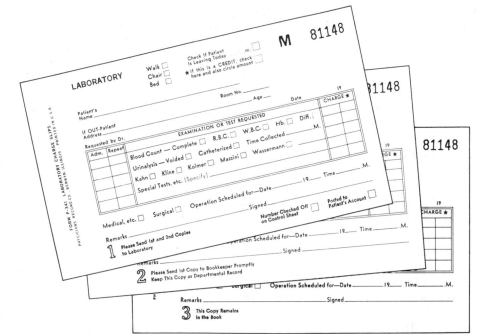

Fig. 6-3. Sample laboratory record forms. (Courtesy Physicians' Record Co.)

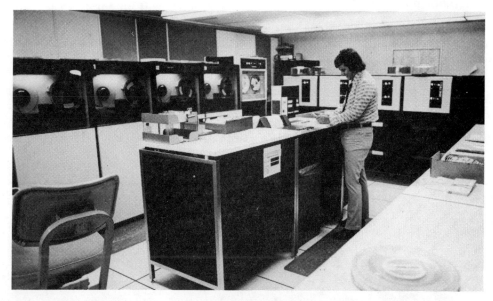

Fig. 6-4. Hospital computer department.

dividual pieces of equipment which operate together to perform certain functions. Without planned and detailed instructions the equipment does nothing at all. The programming, or the "machine-understandable" instructions, is the important part of any computer system. Let's look further into computers and the tasks they are able to perform.

On a magnetic tape or disc there are thousands of magnetic points. We can make these points electrically positive or negative and we can return to the point repeatedly and read this plus or minus condition. We generally refer to the + or − as 0 or 1 or Yes or No. Using this information we can

work out a code. Each of these single points of electric charge is called a bit. These bits are organized into 6 or 8 bit "words" called bytes. The information that is coded in a series of bits or +/− units is called binary (2 units).

Using binary code we can make the bytes represent numbers or words. With these bytes, we are able to translate spoken words and whole numbers into electrical impulses that can be stored on the tapes or discs. We can then establish certain electrical patterns that can be recognized and we can scan the tape or disc for a name or number. Thus, we are able to store data in the form of names or numbers and we can later retrieve the information when we want it. Fortunately, this process can be extremely rapid and we can "search" through many thousands of names and numbers in a fraction of a second.

Other devices that work to help us are the gates that permit us to decide what to do with information. These gates are electronic devices that allow us to retrieve information when two factors (electric signals) are both present. The AND type of gate allows information to pass when two characteristic signals or facts are both present. The OR gate allows either of two signals to pass. The NOR gate passes all information that contains neither one of two signals. Other combinations are possible. Thus, by the use of selective gates we can sort information and retrieve only the kind of information we want. When we apply these capabilities of storing information in binary code and selectively retrieving it, we have the essential features of data storage and retrieval.

Programming

Obviously, the setting up of the code and the instructions for this process becomes a science. We call this science "programming." Programmers are the people who are especially trained to converse with the computers by reducing the written or spoken words to machine-understandable code. Short cuts have been developed in terms of computer languages that translate whole words or expressions into binary code without the painful detail of translating each letter and number into many bits. These different languages are designed for different purposes. ASCI, Cobol, and Fortran are some of the different languages in common use. As systems become more sophisticated, more of the programming is being done by manufacturers, and many systems that are in use do not require that the operator know anything about programming.

Computers are really a system composed of several components or pieces of hardware (Fig. 6-5). The Central Processing Unit, or CPU, is usually a single piece of equipment that contains some storage called buffer, and all of the various circuits that instruct the computer to search, select and compare bits of information. The gates are in this area. There is usually a separate disc or tape storage unit where information is stored. This is the computer's memory. Some device must be available to enable us to "talk" to the computer, telling it to hunt, select, compare, etc. These units are called I/O or input/output devices. This is usually a teletype unit or a keyboard with a television type of screen on which answers appear. These screens are cathode ray tubes or CRTs. We may communicate with the computer in other ways, of course.

For example, to input information we may put data in code form onto punch cards, and card readers can very rapidly read the information into the

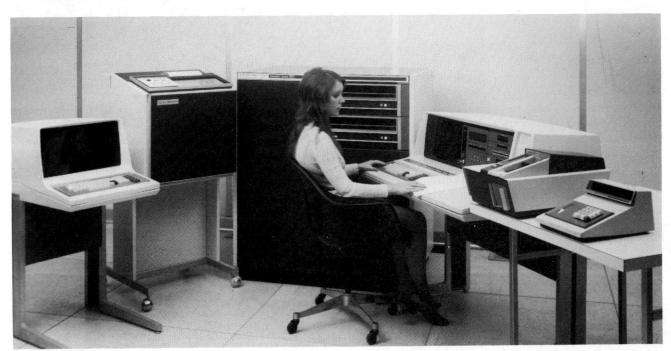

Fig. 6-5. Computer equipment set-up. (Courtesy Spear Medical System, Division of Beckman, Dickinson and Co.)

computer's memory. We may also punch information into punch tape, using a specially equipped teletypewriter. Then a tape reader can read the tape and put the data into storage in the computer's memory. Some types of laboratory equipment, such as analyzers, may give the computer electrical signals. An interface translates the electrical information into meaningful numbers. Usually a PID is also present which allows the operator to put Patient Identification into the computer to match up with the analytical data. When an analyzer or other device feeds information continuously to the computer in this fashion, we say the device is "on line." If the computer accepts such signals interspersed with other activities, we say it is "time sharing."

In order to get information out of the computer, high speed line printers are usually used. These devices can print reports at very high speed and the format of the printed report can be organized in the most readable form. Various other types of printers and cathode ray tube arrangements are also available.

The whole computer system, then, may consist of a central processing unit along with any of several memory units, various sorts of input and output units, such as teletypes, CRTs, card readers, magnetic tape readers, and punch tape readers. Sometimes, various of these elements may be combined so that the over-all system may vary.

Functions of Computers

The functions for which the computer system is designed may be extremely varied also. As we have seen, we can store data, recall them selectively, choose the information on the basis of its characteristics, such as "greater than," "less than," "either," "either/or." Some systems, called analog computers, are designed to accept electrical signals and judge between their amplitude. These analog computers can be designed to solve such complex problems as square roots, log values, and statistical analysis.

From the facts we have just discussed, it is easy to see that computers can be designed to serve many purposes. It is easy to conclude that they can do almost anything and that all we need to do is get a great big computer and let it do everything. This, alas, is easier said than done, since each step along the way is complex enough. When we try to consolidate too many of these functions in one giant step, the resulting system may get to be too cumbersome to work effectively.

Someone has said that there is nothing that can be conceived by the mind that cannot be done through engineering if enough money is available. Putting a man on the moon is a testament to the validity of the statement. That endeavor did require an enormous amount of money, however. The same is true of computer systems. The concept of performing very large numbers of operations by computer is certainly valid. The more complex the operation becomes, the more expensive it is and the more the problems multiply. Let us consider some of the problems in medicine that have been solved by computers and also consider the problems involved.

Hospital Applications

Collection of billing information is a large job in any hospital since charges come from such places as laboratory, pharmacy, x-ray, physical therapy, nursing, central services, etc. Many of these single charges are small and are made for services that require a great deal of explanation. All of these charges are made to individual patients, each of whom has a separate identification number. It is possible to set up a file in the computer that consists of all of the charges being made to one patient, and the file can be recognized by his identification (ID) number. The various services can be given code numbers. Thus the ID #364110 charged 70615 may simply mean that John Davis, who is patient #364110 was charged $10.00 for a blood sugar test, which is code #70615.

70 = Laboratory

6 = Chemistry

15 = Blood Sugar

The entire number tells the computer that the charge is $10.00. Using the time-honored system of paper charge tickets, several hundred charge tickets go to make up the patient's bill. There is much work involved in making out these slips, carrying them to a central billing office, and separating, sorting, posting and filing them. Errors are easy to make as some slips are lost, some are unreadable, some human errors are made, etc. Fifteen percent of the charges to the patient are lost during the manual processing, according to widely accepted estimates. Many of the problems of a manual system can be eliminated by the use of computers and large amounts of paper work are also eliminated in this way. Before we rush wildly to buy a computer, however, let us think about various other aspects of the problem.

Information does not flow effortlessly into the computer in most cases. Some billing document is still usually present and someone has to put the data into the computer by teletype, punch cards, or paper tape. Human errors can still be made during this step. There is also the problem of system failure. When the computer goes down, all records are momentarily lost as certainly as if the lights in the storage vault were turned out. On some occasions, the entire record can be erased from the computer's memory and some "hard copy" record, or hand written record has to be maintained to back up the computer storage. ((Fortunately, techniques have been pretty well developed to keep this sort of thing from happening.) Sometimes the process of recording or retrieving information in usable form may become so complicated that we can spend much time and effort in resolving program problems. Very complex programs have a way of developing "bugs" or errors because of the very complexity of the coding problems.

At the same time, one must remember that, thanks to the orderly classifying process of coding, it is possible to retrieve much information that would be very hard to get by the old system of paper slips. For example, if a blood sugar is coded as we have suggested above, we can retrieve all laboratory charges by getting all 70,000 numbers and we can count blood chemistry tests by counting all 70,600 numbers and a total of all 70,615 charges will tell us the total number of blood sugar tests done in a given time period. By the same system we can pick out the number of male patients, Smiths, 16 year olds, blondes, etc. This sort of information may be very helpful but we need to remember that this is not what we set out to get and that it may not be of any monetary value to know how many 16-year-old, blue-eyed, blonde Smiths were admitted in 1972. This is to say that we need to be certain that the attractive features of the system are the characteristics that we need and can afford to pay a considerable amount of money to get.

Medical Information

Besides collecting charge information, the computer system can be used in many other ways. One of the most promising ways would seem to be the passing of information from place to place. For example, if a nurse could simply tell the computer that a patient was to have an x-ray of the chest, a blood count, and a 5 grain aspirin every 4 hours, the radiology department could receive a request

on its printer or CRT, the pharmacy could package the aspirin (Fig. 6-6), and the laboratory would start the blood count (Fig. 6-7). The idea of this

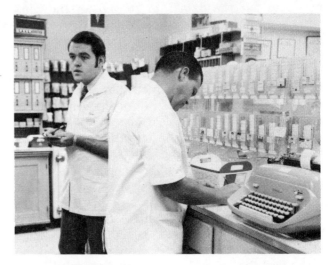

Fig. 6-6. Hospital pharmacy.

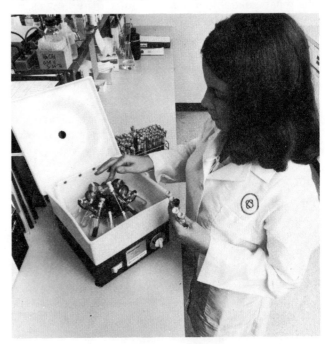

Fig. 6-7. A technician loads blood samples into a blood-cell counting machine. (Courtesy Damon Corp.)

simple, direct system is beautiful. We call this arrangement a Total Information System. It presupposes, however, that every department and every nursing unit has its own computer terminal. Initially, this would be a very large investment. If it were completely trouble free and if it worked immediately upon installation, it might well be worth the price. This is not always the case, however, and few hospitals have used their own funds to install this very sophisticated system yet. It will very probably become practical soon as hardware and programming problems are solved and as mass-produced equipment becomes less expensive.

Some hospitals have gone to very sophisticated medical records systems in which the entire patient's chart, including I.D., doctors' orders, reports, and nursing notes are stored in the computer. Again, the systems are very expensive and there are problems. In medico-legal cases, there is no written and signed doctor's order as evidence, and courts are sometimes unwilling to recognize the computer document as legal evidence since any teletypewriter could be made to produce a similar document in a few minutes. It cannot be denied that a computerized patient record would save much time, effort and storage. The cost and these as yet unsolved problems almost eliminate this use of computers at the present time.

Computers can take electrical signals from analytical instruments and convert them into real numbers. With these numbers they can solve some types of analytical problems. Thus the analysis of a series of blood samples being tested for several components can be recorded, diagnostic information can be deduced, and the error of the analyzer can be predicted. A computer used in this way to monitor one piece of equipment and process its output would be called a "dedicated computer" since all of its functions are dedicated to one purpose. Computers can do this sort of job reasonably well even though some technical problems occasionally arise. The cost is relatively low since the system can be small and only one or two terminals are needed. One job of this sort that can be done rather simply and economically by computers is the interpretation of electrocardiogram tracings. While it is still necessary for a cardiologist to examine unusual records, much time-consuming measuring and interpretation is avoided by using a rather simple computer.

Management Applications

The inventory and ordering of supplies can be expedited, in most cases, through use of the computer. There is still a rather considerable amount of work involved in keeping the computer files current. It is probably no more difficult than keeping hard copy records. Reports and orders are undoubtedly much easier to obtain.

Scheduling, which is a chronic problem in hospitals, can be simplified by the use of a computer.

It is able to evaluate the various possible solutions to complicated situations more quickly than a person could do it. It does not solve human problems of unexpected absences or overloads and some effort must be expended in programming. It may provide some small measure of satisfaction to the harried manager in that it provides something to blame for problems for which there are no easy solutions.

The bed census and bed assignments have been computerized in many hospitals. This system undoubtedly can save some time and prevent errors. Like most problems, there is much more detail to room assignment than is apparent to the outsider, and the computer must be told many details in order to function properly. Less time may be saved than one might suppose but statistics can be produced much more quickly and accurately when they are needed.

When computers are used in the hospital, the chances are that very little actual time will be saved. In fact, the total number of payroll hours expended for any particular function often actually increases. The cost, including lease of equipment, will almost certainly be at least as high as the cost of the manual operation. The value of a computer system is almost always in the improved management capability it provides. It is almost always possible to get a much clearer analysis of any situation by intelligently harvesting the appropriate data from the computer's memory. These summaries can be called up very rapidly at almost any time if the programming has been properly done.

A chronic problem in management is the lack of good, recent and reliable information on which to make a judgment. Where this is the case, the computer is worth its cost. Most often, however, the system is installed to save time, reduce payroll, etc., and this objective is elusive, as we have already emphasized. At the same time, the improvement in management capability that is achieved may be more sorely needed than the manager realizes and he may come out of his traumatic experiences with computers looking better than he had hoped.

Types of Hardware

In general, the hardware produced by various manufacturers works in the same way and uses the same basic principles. There is some difference in reliability, versatility, etc., but these factors possibly vary as much between different models as between producers. The really significant factors are the programming details and the ability of the company to maintain its equipment. Most hospitals cannot afford the costs of total programming of a computer system. Many systems have some of the necessary programs prepared or the producer will undertake a great deal of the programming detail. Some systems are completely programmed so that the operator simply puts in the required information in the prescribed format and asks for information in the established manner. The company that sells the system undertakes to keep programs up to date and provide all maintenance. This sort of installation would be called a turn-key system. Unless the hospital has programming help available or is prepared to get heavily involved in programming, there may be considerable advantage to a turn-key operation. It is initially more expensive but should be more reliable.

The size of the system is important. Storage capability can usually be increased fairly easily. The speed with which information can be made accessible, when storage is near capacity, is a very important performance characteristic. If the system has several terminals this access speed will probably be slower when all terminals are in use. Judgments about such characteristics must be made by someone who has experience and knowledge. The manager would do well to cultivate a healthy, informed skepticism about expensive computer systems even though a smoothly operating computer can be of great value to the operation.

In Figs. 6-8, 6-9 and 6-10, laboratory computer records are shown. Fig. 6-8 is part of a cumulative summary of all of the hematology reports on a patient during his hospital stay. Fig. 6-9 is a laboratory work list that shows the technician in the hematology section what work to expect and gives sample numbers for all specimens. Fig. 6-10 shows the type of labels that are generated to identify samples that are to be drawn.

The Status-I Laboratory Based Computer System

The group of pictures (Fig. 6-11) shows the component parts of a special computer used for one specific function or department. This system is designed to accumulate all of the reports coming from the laboratory and put them together in the form of "summary laboratory reports" which include all tests done during the patient's admission. Summary reports may be called up and read from the CRT screen or printed out on the high speed line printer. The system provides very fast access to all patient information, organization of blood collection lists, work lists for each laboratory department and work station, identification of abnormal test results, and other related efficiencies.

The component parts of the system shown in Fig. 6-11 are:

A. Central Processing Unit or CPU, where all information is stored and where specific data processing functions take place.

B. Input-Output Terminal or I/O, which enables the operator to communicate with the

Fig. 6-8. Laboratory computer record—cumulative summary of hematology tests.

```
SMITH, JOHN          ID-694824      CUMULATIVE SUMMARY   3/ 9/74-10:23  PAGE  01

RM  DISCHARGED  SEX M   DOB 07/12/1951  ADM  2/18/74  DR  HALL


HEMATOLOGY      UNITS    NORMALS      2/28    2/19
                         LOW-HIGH     12:36   11:25

WHITE BLD CT   THOUS. 04.8 10.8    03.9 @   07.5
RED BLD CNT.   /MC MM. 4.10 5.50   3.56 @   2.24 @
HEMOGLOBIN     GMS.   13.0 17.0    10.4 @   06.6 @
HEMATOCRIT     %      39.0 51.0    29.8 @   19.8 @
MCV INDEX      UCUBE  081. 101.    085.     086.
MCH INDEX      UUG    27.0 35.0    29.7     29.9
MCHC INDEX     %      32.0 36.0    35.0     34.0
STABS          %      00.0 05.0    00.0     00.0
NEUTROPHILS    %      050. 075.    079. @   082. @
LYMPHOCYTES    %      24.0 40.0    12.0 @   12.0 @
MONOCYTES      %      02.0 10.0    03.0     04.0
EOSINOPHILS    %      00.0 05.0    06.0 @   02.0
BASOPHILS      %      00.0 02.0    00.0     00.0
ANISOCYTES                         SLIGHT   NONE
POIKILOCYTES                       SLIGHT   SLIGHT
POLYCHROMAT                        OCC      OCC
MACROCYTES                         NONE     NONE
MICROCYTES                         NONE     NONE
STIPPLING                          NONE     NONE
PLATLET APP                        ADEQ     ADEQ
ADD COMMENTS                       NONE     NONE
SPEC NUMBER           000. 999.    184.     750.
```

```
3/ 9/74-16:16 *01   MODEL S      * STATUS I -WORKLIST-      TECH:    PAGE:  0001

                              WBC   RBC   HGB   HCT   MCV   MCH   MCHC
                              I     I     I     I     I     I     I     I
                              I     I     I     I     I     I     I     I
                              I----I----I----I----I----I----I----I----I
                              I     I     I     I     I     I     I     I
                              I     I     I     I     I     I     I     I
                              I----I----I----I----I----I----I----I----I
0083   696314                 I     I     I     I     I     I     I     I
FAJARDO, AIDA                 I     I     I     I     I     I     I     I
     TIME                     I----I----I----I----I----I----I----I----I
0245   696190                 I     I     I     I     I     I     I     I
ARMSTRONG, ROBERT H. IXXXXIXXXXI   I     IXXXXIXXXXI   I
     TIME                     I----I----I----I----I----I----I----I----I
0277   691591                 I     I     I     I     I     I     I     I
JEFFCOAT, FLORENCE EIXXXXIXXXXI    I     IXXXXIXXXXI   I
     TIME                     I----I----I----I----I----I----I----I----I
0282   696244                 I     I     I     I     I     I     I     I
TUCKER, WADE         IXXXXIXXXXI   I     IXXXXIXXXXI   I
     TIME                     I----I----I----I----I----I----I----I----I
0284   696421                 I     I     I     I     I     I     I     I
MACFARLANE, LAVILLA I I       I     I     I     I     I     I
     TIME                     I----I----I----I----I----I----I----I----I
0306   696429                 I     I     I     I     I     I     I     I
STOREY, JAMES        IXXXXIXXXXIXXXXI   IXXXXIXXXXIXXXIXXXXI
     TIME                     I----I----I----I----I----I----I----I----I
0411   691591                 I     I     I     I     I     I     I     I
JEFFCOAT, FLORENCE E I        I     I     I     I     I     I
     TIME                     I----I----I----I----I----I----I----I----I
0414   696345                 I     I     I     I     I     I     I     I
PAINTER, LUCY E.     IXXXXIXXXXIXXXXI   IXXXXIXXXXIXXIXXXXI
     TIME                     I----I----I----I----I----I----I----I----I
0416   696408                 I     I     I     I     I     I     I     I
FELDER, GAY M.                I     I     I     I     I     I     I     I
     TIME                     I----I----I----I----I----I----I----I----I
0417   696201                 I     I     I     I     I     I     I     I
REISE, JOHNATHAN C.  I I      I     I     I     I     I     I
     TIME                     I----I----I----I----I----I----I----I----I
0420   695645                 I     I     I     I     I     I     I     I
HEDGES, NORMAN P.    IXXXXIXXXXI   I     IXXXXIXXXXI   I
     TIME                     I----I----I----I----I----I----I----I----I
0502   695259                 I     I     I     I     I     I     I     I
LINN, STEVEN                  I     I     I     I     I     I     I     I
     TIME                     I----I----I----I----I----I----I----I----I
0531   695929                 I     I     I     I     I     I     I     I
HAMMOND, SIDNEY               I     I     I     I     I     I     I     I
     TIME                     I----I----I----I----I----I----I----I----I
0811   696014                 I     I     I     I     I     I     I     I
POWELL, ADDIE M.             I     I     I     I     I     I     I     I
     TIME                     I----I----I----I----I----I----I----I----I
0957   696006                 I     I     I     I     I     I     I     I
GLENN, GLADIE S.     IXXXXIXXXXI   I     IXXXXIXXXXI   I
     TIME                     I----I----I----I----I----I----I----I----I
1112   696212                 I     I     I     I     I     I     I     I
SMITH, LUCILLE       IXXXXIXXXXIXXXXI   IXXXXIXXXXXIXXXXI
     TIME                     I----I----I----I----I----I----I----I----I
1203   695849                 I     I     I     I     I     I     I     I
PEELING, ROY K.      IXXXXIXXXXI   I     IXXXXIXXXXI   I
     TIME                     I----I----I----I----I----I----I----I----I
```

Fig. 6-9. Laboratory computer work lists.

```
3/ 9/74-16:16 *01   MODEL S      * STATUS I -WORKLIST-      TECH:    PAGE:  0002

                              WBC   RBC   HGB   HCT   MCV   MCH   MCHC
2222   694855                 I     I     I     I     I     I     I     I
DARRAH, CURTIS R.    IXXXXIXXXXI   I     IXXXXIXXXXI   I
     TIME                     I----I----I----I----I----I----I----I----I
2363   694980                 I     I     I     I     I     I     I     I
HUDSON, LUCILLE M.            I     I     I     I     I     I     I     I
     TIME                     I----I----I----I----I----I----I----I----I
2699   694460                 I     I     I     I     I     I     I     I
BENBOW, MOSES        IXXXXIXXXXI   I     IXXXXIXXXXI   I
     TIME                     I----I----I----I----I----I----I----I----I
                              I     I     I     I     I     I     I     I
                              I     I     I     I     I     I     I     I
                              I----I----I----I----I----I----I----I----I
                              I     I     I     I     I     I     I     I
                              I     I     I     I     I     I     I     I
                              I----I----I----I----I----I----I----I----I
                              I     I     I     I     I     I     I     I
                              I     I     I     I     I     I     I     I
                              I----I----I----I----I----I----I----I----I
                              I     I     I     I     I     I     I     I
                              I     I     I     I     I     I     I     I
                              I----I----I----I----I----I----I----I----I
                              I     I     I     I     I     I     I     I
                              I     I     I     I     I     I     I     I
                              I----I----I----I----I----I----I----I----I
                              I     I     I     I     I     I     I     I
                              I     I     I     I     I     I     I     I
                              I----I----I----I----I----I----I----I----I
```

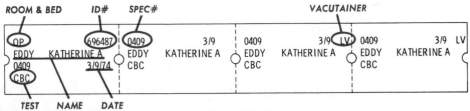

Fig. 6-10. Type of labels used to identify samples.

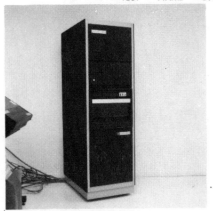

A. Central processing unit. (Courtesy Coulter Electronics, Inc.)

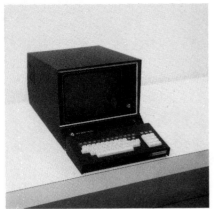

B. I/O terminal. CRT with keyboard.

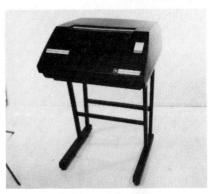

C. High speed line printer.

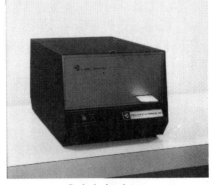

D. Label printer.

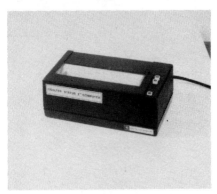

E. Exception printer.

Fig. 6-11. Component parts of a special computer.

computer. This unit is a Cathode Ray Tube (CRT) with a keyboard similar to that of a typewriter. In addition to letters and numbers the keyboard has keys for specific operations or processes that the computer can perform.

C. High Speed Line Terminal, which prints out reports, lists, etc.

D. Label Printer, which prepares labels for all specimens and prints them in the sequence in which blood is to be collected.

E. Exception Printer, which prints out all abnormal results for immediate review by qualified personnel.

Not pictured is Patient Identification Interface for on-line instruments (often called a PID Box). This device allows the operator to tell the computer which patient's sample is being analyzed.

Review Questions

1. Why are computers needed in hospitals?

2. What is a bit? A byte? A CPU?

3. What functions can computers serve in hospitals?

4. What problem causes computers to be questionable for use in preparing medical records?

5. How do we communicate with computers?

6. How do you think a computer might help a manager?

Physical Resources:
Repair and Maintenance

We have said that management is the art of getting the most done with the resources that are available. Aside from personnel, the manager's principal resource is the physical plant and equipment. This may vary from a small space and a few simple devices and supplies to a sizable area with a great deal of sophisticated equipment. Some generalities apply in all cases.

Arrangement of Space

Functional arrangement of work space is very important, whether it is the top of your desk or a 10,000 square foot warehouse. Efficiency experts are paid to study your operation and recommend the proper arrangement of your affairs. You should be your own expert since you know more about your operation than anyone else. This does not mean that experts cannot help you. You need only to be very objective and take the time to think things through. Watch carefully as you and other people work. Look for delays that occur when supplies are not conveniently close. Look for lost time in going after things, reaching, opening and closing, getting up from your desk to get or put away items that could be within reach.

Traffic Patterns

Time and motion studies do not always have to be technical to show significant loss of time in many instances. Floor plans, including work areas, storage, and control points, need to be arranged to correspond to the flow of work. Traffic patterns should be studied to avoid spots where people must wait, cross in front of others, or interrupt others' activities. When concentration is required and when noise and distraction may add to errors, these activities should be shielded from areas of physical activity and heavy traffic. Sound deadening materials, such as screens, floor mats, draperies or even soft-texture bulletin boards, may help reduce noise levels. Signs restricting unnecessary traffic in work areas and arrangement of desks and tables to discourage short-cuts through work areas can reduce confusion. Even the arrangement of lighting and details of decoration may subtly affect flow-patterns, areas of concentration, mood and, incidentally, noise levels.

Cleanliness and Order

It is impossible to manage an operation effectively if it is not orderly. You may feel that you can throw things about and know just where they are, and two or three people may be able to work together this way with some semblance of efficiency but it is not likely that the most work gets done in the least time. A little time spent in arrangement of supplies and inventory, cleaning and arranging work areas, and discarding waste material is more than offset by the time you can save. Aside from the obviously improved ease of finding things, the cleanliness and order have psychological value. People feel more like working and achieving when their surroundings are clean, orderly, and pleasant. Everyone enjoys working in an area he is proud of. It is hard to be proud of a work station that is ankle deep in dirty paper towels and cigarette butts. Dirty windows, smudged paint around doors, cluttered desks and counters, and overflowing wastebaskets reflect an attitude of carelessness and a lack of pride. When an area is extremely busy and crowded, as most hospitals are, it is very hard to avoid the appearance of clutter. Still, the efforts expended in cleaning and improving appearances is usually time well spent.

Inventory

At the present time, hospitals are beginning to experience all sorts of shortages in every conceivable sort of supplies. This is probably a blessing in disguise in some ways. We have become careless and wasteful and, in many cases, improvident. For some poorly defined cost we seem to think we can correct any lack of materials, so why worry? One of the major causes of inefficiency in the hospital is the occasional lack of appropriate supplies. The lack may be from waste, failure to provide substitutes for such contingencies, or storage at the wrong place. All of this may be improved because of current shortages. As we find replacement of wasted supplies becoming more difficult, measures will be taken to avoid needless loss. More attention will be given to adequate inventory levels and we will possibly be more conscious of defective merchandise that decreases workable inventories.

We should surely start to plan some substitutes for items that are hard to get and thought should be given to procedural changes that these substitutions might necessitate. It is very damaging to be caught in the position of not being able to render service because of the temporary lack of supplies or the malfunction of routine equipment. Each instance of this sort is clearly remembered but normal or even superior service is taken for granted. Particularly in health care, there is little patience with service lapses. Make every effort to avoid such situations.

Plan for Contingencies

If you spend a little time working on contingency planning you may be able to avoid considerable embarrassment even when supply and equipment problems are at their worst. All personnel should be trained to minimize service problems. All too often an aide or secretary will rush into an examining room and exclaim, "We're all out of Ace bandages. I don't know what they expect us to do!" The patient promptly goes into hysterics assuming he'll just have to bleed to death since there is no alternative. Problems of service should never be discussed around the patient and if they are inadvertently mentioned should be minimized. The patient is entitled to reasonable confidence in his treatment and the doctor should not have to be involved in details of supply and equipment unless it will affect what he must do. Setting up inventory records, such as the form for syringes and needles shown on Table 7-1 is one very good, and relatively simple, way to prevent sudden shortages of supplies.

Care of Equipment

One of the manager's largest problems is maintenance of equipment. Many large equipment

Table 7-1. Syringe and Needle Inventory Work Form

Item	Average Use Per Week	Time Needed to Obtain After Requisition (Weeks)	Per Week × Weeks Required	Safety Margin	Lower Inventory Level	Upper Inventory Level = Lower Limit + Reasonable Storage
10 ml syringe	65	4	260	65	325	500
5 ml syringe	80	4	320	80	400	600
1 ml syringe	20	4	80	20		125
22 g × 1 needle	150	2	300	150	450	1000
25 × ½″	125	2	250	100	350	500

After this reasoning process is done, inventory cards might be set up showing the lower and upper inventory limits for each item. Each time supplies are received, the cards are up-dated to show the new level. As items are withdrawn the cards are corrected. When the amount on hand falls below the lower inventory level, enough are ordered to bring stocks to the upper inventory level. This level should be sensible. It is expensive to carry needlessly large inventories but imprudent to let them get too low.

systems are involved in any sizeable hospital. There are analyzers, patient monitors, fluoroscopes, computers, air handlers, emergency generators, laundry equipment, distillation equipment, and many more large and complex items representing a total investment of millions of dollars in many cases (Fig. 7-1). Many of these devices are essential to effective patient care.

The addition of this sort of equipment is part of the revolution in hospital care that has recently occurred. We have been slow to realize the problems involved in maintenance and repair. During the past 10 years hospital managers have had very difficult times with expensive and critical pieces of equipment that no one but the factory representative (a thousand miles away) could re-

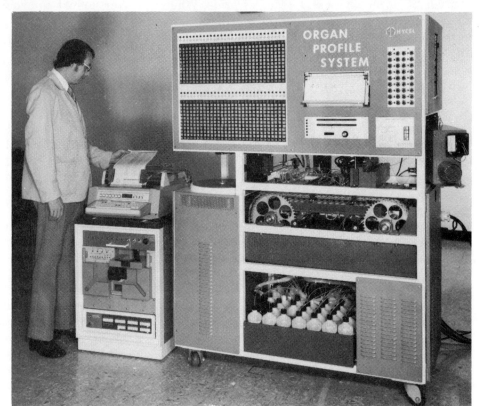

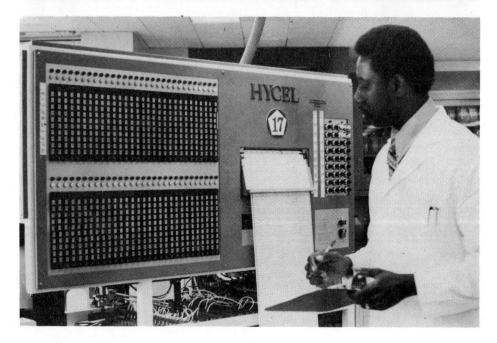

Fig. 7-1. Large automated equipment found in many major medical centers. (Courtesy Hycel, Inc.)

pair. This became such a serious concern that training programs were initiated for medical repairmen; companies were formed to provide repair services, and many large manufacturers lost a great deal of money and reputation because of their failure to provide adequate repairs.

The investments are so large and the problems so critical that it is imperative that adequate maintenance and repair be planned for any reasonable contingency wherever major equipment is in use. These back-up plans and activities usually take place on about four different levels.

Level of Maintenance

1. Certain maintenance steps, adjustments and small repairs are the responsibility of the operator of the equipment. Adequate training of the operator is a critical step that is often omitted. Many companies have special training classes or will send a factory trained representative to the hospital to do this training (Fig. 7-2). A careless or poorly trained operator can cause serious problems that make good equipment effectively useless in spite of good repair support. Maintenance routines must be established and made a matter of regular record. The operator must have access to the factory repair personnel to learn as much as he can about problems that occur. Of course, the operator must be sufficiently knowledgeable and intelligent to understand his equipment. It is poor economy to buy or lease a $100,000 analyzer and send a high school dropout to operate it because the salesman said it was simple. Few salesmen can resist telling you that "A 10 year old boy could operate it!"

   Most hospital equipment concerned with patient care needs to be in the hands of people who thoroughly understand the theoretical and practical aspects of its operation. All calibration checks, maintenance checks and procedures, and other operating data should be filed or posted near the equipment where you and the factory repair man can find and understand them. Do not allow the operator to establish a monopoly on the machine's operation and care. He must be encouraged to take pride in its operation and should derive considerable satisfaction from doing his job well. At the same time, he should not be able to blackmail you because no one else understands his equipment. Even if you have the highest confidence in him, he could have an accident, get sick, or get a better job.

2. The second level of maintenance is usually the supervisor over the actual operator of the system. This is likely to be the person who made the commitment to buy or lease the equipment and he probably has a pretty good idea of its purpose and some idea about what it should be able to do. The decisions concerning maintenance and repair are in

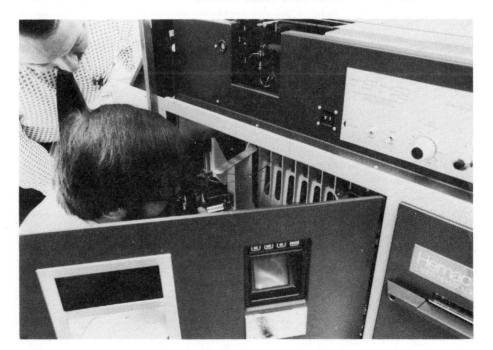

Fig. 7-2. Factory trained representative instructing operator on how to adjust the Hemac™ 630L, Laser hematology counter. (Courtesy Damon Corp.)

his hands. He may have some technical expertise with the equipment and may do some repair or maintenance or he may simply refer the problem to the appropriate person or agency. In small remote areas this person may be the ultimate "Mr. Fixit" or he may simply make the necessary judgment about the next step that should be taken. If he is effective he should have the best idea about what constitutes reasonable service from the system and should react accordingly.

3. The next level of care in most cases is the hospital's in-house electronic repair capability. Some large hospitals have a very complete, very competent repair crew which has been factory trained on many systems. Others may have little more than a handyman. If there is a quantity of sophisticated instrumentation, the employment of one or more good electronics men is probably an excellent investment. A number of schools now graduate several two-year and four-year medical electronics repair men each year and some of the major manufacturers of equipment have started programs for training them on their particular brand of equipment.

4. The final level of repair and maintenance is the factory repair man or representative. The producers of many major hospital systems have begun to realize that the reputation of their equipment is, in large measure, dependent on their repair and maintenance.

Computer companies, as part of their lease arrangement, may actually station a man permanently in the hospital to guarantee that there is no unreasonable down-time or other problems. Other companies provide a year of warranty (Fig. 7-3) and sell a maintenance agreement to the user after the warranty period is finished (Fig. 7-4). Still other companies do repair and maintenance on an hourly basis only. All of these companies have much to lose if their systems fail to perform satisfactorily, because if they fail, reputations are damaged. The loss of only a few sales of very expensive systems can be very costly to the manufacturer.

Most manufacturers of major equipment provide a fairly standard maintenance and repair contract under which they guarantee to check and calibrate the equipment at stated times and to provide repair service. Repairs may be included in the contract price or may be guaranteed at a minimal cost. The price of these contracts varies a great deal, depending upon what is guaranteed, the repair experience with the equipment and, sometimes, upon the distance of the hospital from the closest repair facility. There is no very easy way to judge whether the contract is a good one because of all of these variables. Five percent of the purchase price per year is about what manufacturers figure warranty and maintenance will cost.

Fig. 7-3. Hycel Service Agreement. (Courtesy Hycel, Inc.)

HYCEL SERVICE AGREEMENT

Customer Name and Address

_____

_____

Description of Equipment

_____

_____

Location of Described Equipment

_____

Hycel Sales Representative

_____

Accepted_____
       (Hycel Officer)

Date_____

Completion of Described Equipment Installation_____
                                   (Date)

THIS AGREEMENT is made and entered into by and between "Customer," whose name and address appears elsewhere on this page, and Hycel, Inc., a Delaware Corporation having its principal place of business at 7920 Westpark Drive, Houston, Texas (hereinafter "Hycel").

SUBJECT TO THE TERMS AND CONDITIONS of this Agreement on the inside page 2 hereof, Hycel agrees to provide and Customer agrees to accept. (1) in the first year commencing with the date of completion of installation of the Described Equipment, free Hycel Expanded Comprehensive Service with its limitless service call availability during the initial three months after such commencement date; and (2) on the anniversary date of such installation, continuance of Hycel Comprehensive Service or, at Customer's option, any one of (a) Hycel Quality Assurance Service, (b) Hycel Standby Service, (c) Hycel On Call Emergency Service, or (d) no Hycel service.

To complete this Hycel Service Agreement, furnish the signature of an authorized representative for Customer:

Signature_____

Date_____

© 1973, HYCEL, INC.

```
HYCEL SERVICE AGREEMENT
STANDARD CONVERSION FORM

This Conversion Notice is to be attached to and becomes a part of that certain HYCEL SERV-
ICE AGREEMENT by and between HYCEL, Inc. and_____
_____("Customer").
The signature of date hereinbelow written is to authorize Hycel to convert the Service in effect
under said HYCEL SERVICE AGREEMENT to:
    □ Hycel Comprehensive Service
    □ Hycel Quality Assurance Service
    □ Hycel Standby Service
    □ Hycel On Call Emergency Service
    (Check Service conversion desired)
Effective upon the anniversary of the commencement date of said HYCEL SERVICE AGREE-
MENT following receipt of this notice of conversion, the monthly charge for the Service to which
conversion is made will be as stated in the HYCEL SERVICE AGREEMENT.

CUSTOMER

By_____
        Authorized Signature

Date_____
```

Fig. 7-4. Hycel Service Agreement standard conversion form. (Courtesy Hycel, Inc.)

Maintenance Contracts

Since there are so many manufacturers, it may be necessary to carry several different contracts. Some companies such as Bendix, Honeywell, and On-Call have proposed to provide repair and maintenance contracts on all kinds of hospital equipment. For small hospitals this type of contract may prove to be a good solution to many problems. For very large hospitals, the "total repair" contract may prove to be impractical for this approach. Several large companies are examining this concept of total maintenance and repair for all hospital equipment but the problems are formidable.

Minor Maintenance

As a part of its biannual inspection of hospitals, the Joint Commission on Accreditation of Hospitals has started to check the calibration and repair records of equipment. For example, the JCAH wants records of the temperature variation of refrigerators, incubators, sterilizers and autoclaves taken over various time periods. Inspectors may ask for proof of the accuracy of fever thermometers and wave-length calibration of spectrophotometers. These may seem to be unusual details for an accreditation inspector to check, but the idea is very sound. Too many of us have assumed that thermometers are always correct, that autoclaves always sterilize, and that distilled water is necessarily pure. These inspections are calling attention to the fact that any of these things may be in error.

Thermometers can be checked against a government certified thermometer or against an electronic thermometer that has been recently calibrated and certified by a reputable meteorology laboratory. Temperature records on blood and drug refrigerators, particularly, should be made occasionally, showing hour to hour variation.

Obsolescence and Deterioration

A considerable problem with modern equipment is obsolescence. New techniques are developing so rapidly that the devices, that were the very best three years ago, may now be of little utility. In spite of all efforts to prevent this kind of problem it occasionally happens to nearly every institution. Another problem is real deterioration of equipment to the point at which the cost of repairs make its continued use unfeasible. In both cases, some judgment must be made about the reasonable time to get rid of it. Adequate records are the only way of deciding when this time has arrived and even this is not always easy.

In the statistical records of the hospital there is usually enough information about procedures performed, records processed, and payroll hours expended to permit some judgment of the efficiency of equipment systems. Technical judgments must also be made, of course. Whether it is reasonable to go from a scanning system in nuclear medicine to a Gamma Camera is a technical decision that must be based on mature consideration of many factors, including the work volume and probable demand for additional tests that could be done. Adequate records and recorded estimates should support this technical judgment, however.

Once the decision has been made that a piece of equipment is obsolete, the disposition of it becomes a problem. If it has any trade-in value, it should probably be traded as soon as possible since each passing month renders it more obsolete. Often it is thought to have some value as a back up method in case the new equipment fails. This idea is generally not realistic. The new equipment will be under warranty for some time and is not likely to fail. After that time, the effort needed to re-initiate the use of the old system would probably solve the problem with the new one. The work done by the old system was probably inadequate in some way or it would not have been retired from service. For all of these reasons it will probably never be used. What does one do with a five-year old device that once cost $30,000? It is hard to throw

```
                         HISTORY  OF  MAINTENANCE                          PAGE  121

                        ON  LABORATORY  EQUIPMENT

                     JANUARY, 1971  THRU  DECEMBER, 1972
```

ITEM NO.	EQUIPMENT NAME	MANUFACTURE	MODEL-NO.	SERIAL-NO.	YR OF PURCH.	YR OF DEPR.	COST OF EQUIPMENT
129	RECORDER	SARGENT	SRL	639004			$.

DATE		MAINTENANCE PERFORMED ON EQUIPMENT	WORK HOURS	PRICE OF PARTS
	43	TOTAL HOURS AND PARTS THRU DECEMBER 1, 1971.	06.6	$ 45.70
12/23/71	23	CLEAN AND OIL THE PEN CARRIAGE SHAFT.	01.0	$ 3.00
	26	OPERATIONAL CHECK.		
	30	CALIBRATION.		
	46	REPLACED THE MOTOR.		
02/21/72	23	CLEAN AND OIL THE PEN CARRIAGE SHAFT.	01.0	$ .00
	26	OPERATIONAL CHECK.		
	46	REPLACED THE MOTOR.		
04/03/72	35	UNABLE TO COMPLETE-LACK OF PARTS OR TEST DATA.	00.0	$ .00
02/21/72	53	PRICE OF PARTS NOT PREVIOUSLY RECORDED.	00.0	$ 4.90
04/14/72	21	LUBRICATION.	01.0	$ .00
	22	LUBRICATE MOTOR.		
	31	TEST AND/OR REPLACE BATTERIES OR MERCURY CELLS.		
04/24/72	35	UNABLE TO COMPLETE-LACK OF PARTS OR TEST DATA.	00.5	$ .00
	61	TEMPORARILY REMOVED FROM SERVICE.		

Fig. 7-5. History of maintenance on laboratory equipment.

Instrument Record

EQUIPMENT: Centrifuge, large

MANUFACTURER & MODEL: Whirlaway, Model Spin-eze

SERIAL #: 05780

PURCHASE DATE: 6/25/68   PRICE: $353.00

WARRANTY: 1 year from 6/25/68 - forms filed

PURCHASED FROM: Scientific Surplus Sales, Atlanta, Ga.

SERVICE AND WARRANTY BY: Same

ACCESSORIES: 1-6 place head cat. #LXP

　　　　　　　6 - 15 ml shields #666

　　　　　　　6 - cushion #666-S

SERVICE ROUTINE: Inspect, rebalance, lubricate and change brushes every

　　　　6 months. Pull motor and check and/or replace bearings every two years.

　　　　Replace wiring and switch after 4 years.

12/28/68 - Balanced, lubricated and inspected. Brushes don't need changing.

　　　Cost - Labor $1.50

6/25/69 - Balanced and lubricated. Brushes badly worn, with one brush wire

　　　dragging on commutator. Brushes replaced. Cost - Labor $1.50 Parts - $1.75

9/25/69 - Sent in for repair. Brushes worn down to contact wire. Commutator

　　　scratched and pitted. Rotor removed and commutator turned down.

　　　Armature coils O.K. Bearings O.K. Brushes replaced. Lubricated,

　　　balanced and checked. Returned to service. Cost - Labor - $12.50

　　　Parts - $1.75 Cumulative repair to date $19.00

Fig. 7-6. Typical instrument record.

it in the trash but this is often about the only solution. Sometimes some parts can be cannibalized from the old system for repairs. Sometimes a dealer in used equipment may be able to buy it for resale. Occasionally one may be able to give or sell such items to a small foreign hospital, a university, or a trade school and take a tax loss. Occasionally these machines may be good for teaching aids. All too often they are junk and one must reluctantly close his eyes and drop the glory of yesteryear into the garbage. How does one decide the useful life span of such equipment for depreciation? It's not easy.

Records of Equipment Repair

If an in-house repair capability exists, detailed records should be established to show how much has been spent on an item, what its reliability is, and what sort of failures occur. The type of repair record that can be kept is shown in Fig. 7-5. This one is kept by computer.

When major equipment is received, the following specific steps are suggested:

1. Check the packing ticket to be sure the equipment and accessories shipped correspond to the original order.

2. Remove all instruction books and materials. Read them carefully and file them where

they are available to anyone who needs them. If they are detailed, reproduce them or request additional copies.

3. Fill out and return the warranty information if applicable.

4. If a factory representative is to install the equipment, wait for him to do it. If you are over-anxious you may cause serious damage.

5. Do not sign equipment over for payment until you are satisfied with its operation.

6. Set up procedures for maintenance and be sure they are followed.

7. Find out what supplies will be needed and set up an inventory and a procedure for replenishing supplies as needed.

8. Fill out an equipment record showing the name of the equipment, serial number, date of purchase, cost and any other pertinent data, such as manufacturer and source of supplies and repair parts (Fig. 7-6).

9. Check to see that all maintenance, repair, breakdown and up-dating is carefully recorded. Do not neglect quality control steps and calibration procedures.

Review Questions

1. How can quiet work areas be maintained?

2. Set up an inventory system for bed rails for a 45 bed ward. These are constantly reused but may need to be sent for repair at times. Assume that two-thirds of the beds might need rails at the same time.

3. What repair and maintenance resources should you, as laundry manager, develop for a large tumbler?

4. Who should make decisions concerning repair? Explain your answer or answers.

5. What records would you keep on an autoclave provided for the preparation of baby formulas?

6. Discuss in class the criteria you would use to decide whether an electric floor polisher should be replaced.

Purchasing and Leasing

Among the most critical challenges faced by administrative and financial managers in the health care field today is the need for capital funds. In 1970, spending for health care stood at $70 billion. There is a projection that $120 billion will be needed by 1980. The Department of Health, Education and Welfare, in rather conservative estimates, indicates that during the next five years close to $20 billion will be needed by hospitals for expansion and modernization of facilities. As a manager in the allied health care field one of your most important problems will be to cope with finances.

Institutions today are faced with increasing needs for highly technical medical equipment that rapidly becomes obsolete. In earlier years, depreciation reserves were often adequate for the replacement of obsolete equipment. But much medical equipment today did not even exist 10 years ago. Moreover, it is no longer uncommon to find that existing equipment requires replacement before it has fully depreciated.

Leasing

Faced with continuing demands on their capital resources, many hospitals have chosen to rent or lease equipment, especially when a high degree of obsolescence or relatively rapid technology change is expected. In the past, when equipment was purchased outright, the cash flow allowed easier payment than is the case today.

There is a widening recognition that it is simply good management to fully reimburse the cost of equipment during its expected useful life. This is one of the major reasons for the growth of leasing of equipment in this counry (Table 8-1).

A question that often comes up is how to define the difference between a lease and a rental. Let us say that a lease builds up equity, which means that part of the payments the consumer makes can be applied toward paying off the cost of the equipment. Thus, the lease is actually considered a conditional sale or an installment purchase by the Internal Revenue Service and third-party reimbursement agencies. Conversely, rental does not imply a build-up of equity; a rental is a payment for the use of equipment. Therefore, rentals fully qualify as operating expenses, the same as payroll, supplies, expendables, and rent.

How To Lease Equipment

The manager's first objective is to decide what type (or types) of equipment to lease. Once that has been decided, the next step is to request the manufacturer's representative or supplier to send a salesman to discuss the matter and have him get in touch with one of the leasing companies in the field that handles the particular equipment in which the institution is interested. Since not all leasing companies have representatives, a contract might be sent directly to the manager, or whoever is authorized to do so, to be signed. Obviously,

Table 8-1. Laboratory Computer Systems Costs—Purchase vs. Leasing.

Outright Purchase Price	Maintenance Per Month	Purchase Plus Maintenance		
		Total Cost In 36 Mo.	Total Cost In 60 Mo.	Total Cost In 96 Mo.
100,000	$ 600	121,600	136,000	157,600
150,000	$ 900	182,400	204,000	236,400
200,000	$1,200	243,200	272,200	315,200
250,000	$1,500	304,000	340,000	394,000

Outright Purchase Price	*Lease Plus Maintenance					
	36 Months		60 Months		96 Months	
	Total Cost	Per Month	Total Cost	Per Month	Total Cost	Per Month
100,000	$136,800	3,800	162,000	2,700	201,600	2,100
150,000	$226,800	6,300	243,000	4,050	302,400	3,150
200,000	$302,400	8,400	324,000	5,400	403,200	4,200
250,000	$378,000	10,500	405,000	6,750	504,000	5,250

*Lease figures are based on the following:

36 Month Lease—$32. per $1,000.
60 Month Lease—$21. per $1,000.
96 Month Lease—$15. per $1,000.

(Courtesy Spear Medical Systems, Division of Beckman, Dickinson and Company, B-D, Waltham, Massachusetts)

the leasing agreement must be studied very carefully by the authorized person and the hospital's legal counsel before it is signed.

When the lease agreement has been returned to the leasing company, the company will check the hospital's or manufacturer's credit and after the credit is approved will issue a purchase order to the supplier. The supplier then invoices the leasing company. The leasing company may request from the hospital an equipment acceptance form to be signed (Fig. 8-1).

The leasing company will not pay the supplier until it receives the signed copy from the institution stating that the equipment is in the hospital, working, and in satisfactory condition. Once this has been completed, the leasing company pays the manufacturer the full invoice price.

It is good management to look for a leasing company that can structure the payments to coincide with the revenues the new equipment will generate. Simply stated, a laboratory that obtains new equipment will generate income for the hospital; however, it may take from six months to one year for the instrument to be used to its full capacity.

The lease might be arranged so that the payments start low and increase as the equipment is put into greater use. It might also be worthwhile to consider a leasing company that has a used equipment resale facility. This service can be a great advantage because it provides the institution with an enormous amount of flexibility in the field of scientific equipment, which has perhaps the greatest obsolescence factor of any in the health care industry.

The question often arises as to whether an institution that rents or leases equipment from a leasing company rather than from a manufacturer directly will be penalized in any way. The answer is no. All leasing companies pass on to their consumers all the benefits that the customer would have received if the institution had bought the equipment outright directly from the manufacturer. Now, this also includes such items as guarantees, warranties, and if the manufacturer offers a training program for employees who use the equipment, the actual training program. The leasing company pays the manufacturer for the equipment on behalf of the institution.

Equipment Acceptance

ΤΓ̈ι

Telco Leasing, Inc.

Lease number

Lease start

Name and address of Lessee

Name and address of equipment supplier

Equipment location if different from above

Person to contact

Supplier's salesman

Phone number

Phone number

Quantity	Description of equipment	Model no. and other identification

Gentlemen:

All of the items referred to above were received by us in good order and condition, and are acceptable to us.

It is understood and agreed that Telco Leasing, Inc. in no way or manner assumes any responsibility, either now or hereafter, for the use, performance, functioning, maintenance or service of the equipment, or for its suitability or adaptability for any particular purpose.

Lessee _____

By _____

Title _____

Date _____

Fig. 8-1. Equipment acceptance form. (Courtesy Telco Leasing, Inc.)

To help make some of the leasing terminology understandable, a glossary of common terms is included at the end of this chapter.

Paying the complete price for new equipment out of savings or profits of the institution may seriously endanger its financial operation. Cash flow is important, and laying out large sums of money for extremely expensive equipment is basically poor management, so it is good to consider the incentives for leasing or renting (Figs. 8-2 and 8-3).

Keep in mind the possibility of hidden costs that may exist in your leasing agreements (Fig. 8-4) and study the agreements very carefully. If at all possible, you should ask more than one leasing company to submit a proposal. Some of the large companies may not offer the consumer the individual attention that a small or less well established company can. However, large leasing companies have the facilities and the manpower to offer the institution many services. Such services usually include the training of persons in the proper use of equipment, and helping managers to choose the kinds of equipment that will be most useful from among the wide range offered.

Small Equipment and Disposables

It is important to consider the same techniques for both small equipment and disposable items. Any kind of material that is needed to run a hospital laboratory, for example, should be thought of as material needed versus cash flow. Not having to tie up capital in areas in which leasing or renting can be used frees that much more money for other needs of the institution.

Cost Analysis

Cost analysis makes it possible to determine what it is costing the hospital for employees, equipment, and other essential items (Table 8-2). Careful analysis might indicate that a piece of leased equipment is not being used in the best way to give a good return on the investment.

For example, a piece of automated equipment for the clinical chemistry laboratory costs $100 a month on the lease contract. Costing out the equipment may show that because of the number of samples that are being run per day, the personnel needed, and the space required to house this equipment, only enough money, or not even

**Hospital Cash Cost Comparison
(Over Five Years)**

Equipment Price=$100,000	Five-Year Rental ($2,050 per mo.)	Lease-Purchase ($2,200 per mo.)	Cash Purchase	Purchase via 5-Year Bank Loan ($2,050 per mo.)
1 Cost Over Five Years	$123,000	$132,000	$100,000	$123,000
2 Depreciation	N.A.	$ 50,000	$ 50,000	$ 50,000
3 Interest	N.A.	$ 32,000	N.A.	$ 26,000
4 Total Expense for Blue Cross/Medicare Reimbursement (1) or (2)+(3)	$123,000	$ 82,000	$ 50,000	$ 76,000
5 Blue Cross/Medicare Reimbursement (60%×4)	$ 73,800	$ 49,200	$ 30,000	$ 45,600
6 Cumulative Net Cash Cost (1)–(5)	$ 49,200	$ 82,800	$ 70,000	$ 80,400

Assumptions: Bank Loan at 8½%
simple interest for 5 years
10-Year Straight Line Depreciation
60% Blue Cross/Medicare Reimbursement

Fig. 8-2. Hospital cash cost comparisons over five years. (Courtesy Telco Marketing Services, Inc.)

Hospital Cash Cost Comparison
(Over Three Years)

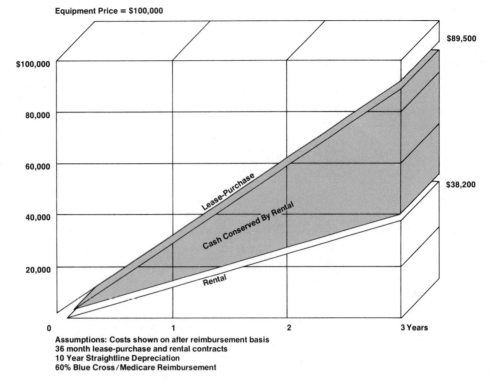

Equipment Price = $100,000

Fig. 8-3. Hospital cash cost comparison over three years. (Courtesy Telco Marketing Services, Inc.)

Assumptions: Costs shown on after reimbursement basis
36 month lease-purchase and rental contracts
10 Year Straightline Depreciation
60% Blue Cross/Medicare Reimbursement

Present Value Cost
Rental vs. Cash Purchase

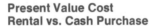

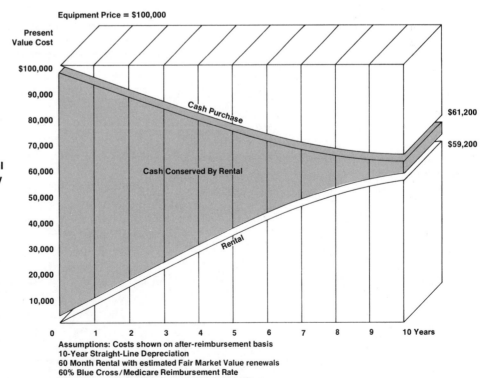

Equipment Price = $100,000

Fig. 8-4. Present value cost rental vs. cash purchase. (Courtesy Telco Marketing Services, Inc.)

Assumptions: Costs shown on after-reimbursement basis
10-Year Straight-Line Depreciation
60 Month Rental with estimated Fair Market Value renewals
60% Blue Cross/Medicare Reimbursement Rate
7% per year present value discount of cash future flows

Table 8-2. Cost Analysis Statistics From 14 Hospitals

# of Hospital Beds	# of Lab Tests	# of Tests per Bed	Annual $$$$$$ Volume of Lab Tests	Average Revenue per Test	# of Lab Personnel	Annual Salaries of Lab Personnel	Average Annual Salary per Lab Personnel	Labor Cost per Test	Annual Lab Salaries % of Annual
420	600,000	1428	1,500,000	2.50	54	418,500	7,750	.70	27.9
555	750,000	1351	2,500,000	3.33	75	570,600	7,600	.76	22.8
517	900,000	1741	2,700,000	3.00	80	640,000	8,000	.71	23.7
425	517,000	1216	1,100,000	2.13	58	349,972	6,034	.68	31.8
500	576,000	1152	2,300,000	3.99	74	599,992	8,108	1.04	26.1
605	800,000	1322	1,800,000	2.25	110	784,960	7,136	.98	43.6
550	1,085,000	1973	1,600,000	1.47	45	439,965	9,777	.41	27.5
330	454,000	1376	1,400,000	3.08	60	450,000	7,500	.99	32.1
526	758,000	1441	1,256,000	1.66	64	620,992	9,703	.82	49.4
340	500,000	1471	1,350,000	2.70	47	524,990	11,170	1.05	38.9
320	250,000	781	1,200,000	4.80	35	364,000	10,400	1.46	30.3
315	400,000	1270	1,080,000	2.70	49	399,987	8,163	1.00	37.0
410	680,000	1659	1,836,000	2.70	60	480,000	8,000	.71	26.1
285	382,000	1340	1,031,400	2.70	48	384,000	8,000	1.01	37.2
ABOVE STATISTICS AVERAGED									
436	618,000	1417	1,618,000	2.62	61	501,954	8,229	.81	31.0
YOUR HOSPITAL									

(Courtesy Spear Medical Systems, Division of Beckman, Dickinson and Company, B-D, Waltham, Massachusetts.)

enough, is brought in to justify the $100-a-month cost. Only through cost analysis is it possible to tell unequivocally whether there is enough income to maintain the equipment and also make a profit (Table 8-3). Cost analysis often provides a stimulus for finding ways to make better use of equipment.

Cost analysis is a time consuming but also a very necessary part of a manager in the allied health field. Many books have been written about cost analysis and many courses on the subject are available. A novice should consider expanding his knowledge by taking a course that explores all avenues of cost analysis.

Let us consider another area for which you as a manager will be responsible, and that is stocking and inventory control.

Inventories of Supplies

To determine how great an inventory of various supplies you should keep you have to find out, first, how much storage space you have and, second, how often you need the item you propose to buy. Stor-

age in any institution is a prime and very costly item, so storage of nonessential materials is wasteful. For example, building up a large inventory of automated analyzer cups just because you can get a good price may not be a wise decision. These cups may occupy space that is needed for some more valuable article that moves out rapidly.

When you are stocking any type of equipment, from small glassware to sheets of paper, you should consider the priority of use. To do this, create a stock ledger that will allow you to follow consumption of the supplies at any time. Most of these ledgers are set up with a code number or letter that will make keeping track of the supply easier. One person should be responsible for keeping the stock ledger. This ledger should list the item, its whereabouts, its code number or letter, and a cutoff number which automatically indicates that reordering is necessary. For example, when the supply gets down to within a limit that you know is absolutely critical, a red tag in the stock room would indicate that immediate reorder is necessary. What is on hand is only the supply needed for one month's work. A yellow tab in the supply room

Table 8-3. A Model Study of a Hospital Laboratory With 400,000 Tests Per Year (Base Test Volume)

Year	(1) # of Tests	(2) Annual Revenue	(3) Lost Charges	(4) Labor Savings	(5) System Savings	(6) System Costs	(7) Net Savings	(8) Net Savings Per Test
5	644,204	1,610,510	48,315	77,304	125,619	300,000	223,817	10.2¢
4	585,640	1,464,100	43,923	70,277	114,100	240,000	158,198	9.3¢
3	532,400	1,331,000	39,930	63,888	103,818	180,000	103,998	8.2¢
2	484,000	1,210,000	36,300	58,080	94,380	120,000	60,180	7.1¢
1	440,000	1,100,000	33,000	52,800	85,800	60,000	25,800	5.9¢
Base	400,000	1,000,000	30,000	48,000	* 78,000	....	....	......

(1) # of tests in base year is 400,000 with a growth rate of 10% per year.
(2) Annual Revenue is assumed at $2.50 per test**.
(3) Lost Charges are based on 3% of annual revenue.
(4) Labor is assumed at $.80 per test with a savings of 15% per year.
(5) System Savings or direct savings due to a laboratory computer is equal to (3) Lost Charges plus (4) Labor Savings.
(6) System Costs assumes a $5000 monthly cost and are cumulative for 60 months.
(7) Net Savings are cumulative each year, i.e., (5) System Savings—System Costs ($60,000/yr) + previous year's Net Savings.
(8) Net Savings per test equals the annual net savings per year divided by the annual test volume.

*Figure appearing in this box is maximum annual expenditure to be made for a computer system if one wishes to show a savings at the end of year one.

**The average revenue of $2.50 per test is assumed to be constant over the 5 years. This figure may increase annually but we are assuming only enough to offset the added cost of labor per test.

(Courtesy Spear Medical Systems, Division of Beckman, Dickinson and Company, B-D, Waltham, Massachusetts).

could be a warning indicating that you are at 25 to 50 percent of your stock. A cross check between a ledger stock item and a shelf indicator provides a double check to keep you from running out of supplies and running into serious problems.

Purchasing

As you progress in the managerial role, several items will become commonplace to you. One of these will be bids. Bids can be made on the state, federal, local, or private level. A bid means you are requesting one or more companies to tell you in writing how much they will charge for a particular item.

Specifications for the particular item are mailed to, let us say, three manufacturers with a request for bids or price quotations for this item. When the bids are returned you can compare them and will then be able to decide logically which company offers the best quality of the merchandise you need at the lowest cost.

If you buy directly from a manufacturer you are eliminating the middle man. If you buy from a large supply house the price will increase because the manufacturer is using that supply house to get the benefit of its distribution capability. The supply house makes its money by charging a higher price than the manufacturer does. Therefore, if you are purchasing material that can be bought from either the manufacturer or a dealer, it is wise to go directly to the manufacturer to save the cost of the approximately 40 percent markup that has been added to the dealer's price to cover his costs. Many dealers have an agreement with the manufacturer that the manufacturer can advertise or sell directly to individual purchasers as well as through the dealer.

Consider quantity buying because it influences the price. If you are going to be needing five cases of pencils or pads of paper for your office, buying one box at a time is more expensive than is purchasing five cases at one time. Supplies like pencils and papers and certain laboratory products do not have an expiration date. So if you have allocated your space properly there should be no difficulty in stock-piling this material when it is on sale. However, when you purchase supplies that have an expiration date, carefully review your situation before you buy. Keep items that require an expiration date separate from the nondated material so you can keep track of the flow of these supplies. Also, it will be to your interest to find out first whether the dealer is willing to take back unused supplies after the expiration date. If such an agreement can be reached you do not have to worry about using up this material within a certain period.

How To Prepare a Bid Request

Following is the information required to fill out a bid request.

1. Date: Enter the date on which you are issuing the bid request.

2. No Later Than: Where it says "no later than" enter the date you think the material must be delivered in order to keep your operation going. Allow a safety margin.

3. Company's Address: Fill in your company's name, which should include zip code and the address to which the material should be delivered.

4. Quantity: Under "quantity" insert the amount of material you require.

5. Item Number: Use catalog number of the company from which you are ordering to correctly identify the items you are requesting. When the company is not the manufacturer, it is wise to use the manufacturer's catalog number to be sure the item bid is equivalent to that ordered. State whether a substitute is acceptable, and specify if samples of the substitution are desired.

6. Description of items ordered: The manufacturer's catalog indicates a description of the material; enter it in this column.

7. You can include in this space a statement indicating that if the company has any questions about your bid someone should call a given number and "ask for Mr. Thompson." Do this in case the catalog from which you ordered the product is now obsolete or the company no longer manufactures it so a representative can let you know and perhaps suggest a replacement.

8. You may wish to specify method and times of delivery, who pays shipping, etc. You may also wish to state that the bid will be judged on an "all-or-none" basis or alternatively on an "item-by-item" basis.

This is all you are basically required to fill out. All bids have terms and conditions on which you and the manufacturer must agree and it is worth your while to read all of the terms and conditions in the bid very closely.

When the bid is returned it should include all of the following:

1. Individually priced items that are legible and easy to read so that you know what price is quoted for the individual items.

2. An authorized company signature which obligates the company to the terms and conditions of the bid.

3. The lower portion of the quotation completely filled in by the bidder. This information will let you know how the material you order is to be shipped and any discounts you may be allowed if you pay within a certain period of time.

You may see no quote next to an item you have requested, which means the company is not able to bid on it for one reason or another. You may have to have two bids from two different companies to complete one order. This is perfectly acceptable and it is easily done. A request for a quotation is not an order, it is asking a supplier to give you a bid on the article you have requested. By sending out several quotations to different manufacturers you are able to ensure not only the best price but also the shortest time in which you can obtain the needed supplies.

Glossary of Leasing Terms

Accelerated Depreciation
Depreciation technique providing for a higher write-down of asset value during early years of asset life. Typical methods are "double declining balance" and "sum of the years' digits."

Accelerated Lease
Lease providing for larger payments early in the term and lower payments later on.

Add-On Interests
Interest used for equal-payment loans or leases, which is expressed as a percentage of original principal. The total charge equals principal times Add-On interest times loan term (in years).

Asset/Expansion
A means of turning fixed assets into cash while retaining the use of the assets.

Balloon Payment
A single relatively large payment at end of lease, rental or loan term, which has the effect of reducing on-going periodic payments.

Book Loss	Loss recorded on company's profit and loss statement when a capitalized asset is sold for less than its book value.
Book Value	The undepreciated balance sheet value of equipment. Does not necessarily have any relationship to fair market value.
Buyout	Transaction in which lessee (user) purchases equipment prior to expiration of lease contract.
Capitalized Asset	An asset appearing on a balance sheet, which is subsequently depreciated.
Compensating Balance	Cash which is required to be left on deposit with lender, generally drawing no interest. A 20% compensating balance is an amount frequently requested by banks. This, in effect, increases the cost of the loan because only 80% of the total loan can be utilized while interest is charged on the total balance.
Compound Interest	Interest calculated on the unpaid (loan or investment) principal balance plus any previously accrued, but unpaid interest.
Conditional Sale	A financing contract in which the user does not receive the asset's title until completion of the contractual payments. This is referred to also as an installment purchase.
Decelerated Lease	Lease providing for lower payments early in the lease term and increased payments later.
Depreciation	Cost or expense arising from planned periodic writedown of book value of capitalized assets.
Fair Market Value	The value of assets as established by what a willing buyer will pay to a willing seller in the open market at a given point in time.
Full Payout Lease	Lease in which the total of all obligated payments equals or exceeds asset cost plus financing charges. Also called a Finance Lease.
Lease	A contract under which the user of assets makes payment for such use over a prescribed period of time and where title remains with the lessor.
Lease/Exchange	A new marketplace for long-term rentals and leases that can help the lessee avoid penalties if he wants to terminate his contract early.
Lease Rate	The periodic charge to a lessee for the use of assets, normally stated as a percent of original asset cost (per month or quarter).
Lessee	User of leased assets.
Lessor	Owner of leased assets.
Net Lease	Lease covering use of assets only. Insurance, maintenance and taxes and other similar obligations are the responsibility of the lessee.
NonPayout Lease	Contract in which the total of all obligated payments is less than original asset cost plus financing charges. This is also called an Operating Lease or rental.
Present Value	The current worth of specific sums of money that is to be received or paid, assuming a given interest rate, or rate of inflation.
Purchase Option	The right that is granted to the lessee by the lessor to purchase the leased assets at a preagreed or negotiated price.
Reimbursement	Payments made by third party agencies (e.g. Blue Cross and Medicare) toward repayment of a provider's operating expenses.
Renewal Option	The right that is granted a lessee at the end of the initial lease term, to renew the lease at preagreed or negotiated rates.

Rental	Payments for the use, rather than ownership, of an asset ("true" lease). Also applied to short-term or "non-payout" contracts.
Residual Value	Value of leased assets at the end of the basic lease term.
Return Option	Option granted lessee to return leased asset to lessor at an agreed future time. Usually it is given without contingent liability.
Sale-Leaseback	Arrangement whereby owner-user of an asset sells it to lessor and leases or rents it back. It will generate cash that is equal to sale price of the asset to the lessor.
Simple Interest	Interest calculated on average unpaid (loan or investment) principal balance over its full term.
Straight Line Depreciation	Depreciation technique providing for equal writedown of asset value each year of the depreciable life of the asset.
Term	The time covered by a lease or rental contract.

*Glossary supplied by Telco Leasing Co., Chicago.

Review Questions

1. Define a "lease."

2. Define "rental."

3. What is meant by "term?"

4. Bids can be made on the state, _____, _____, _____ or _____ levels.

5. Define Lease/Exchange.

6. List the eight items necessary to fill out a bid.

7. Do all bids have terms or conditions? Explain.

8. Does an authorized signature have to appear on the bid?

chapter

9

Finances

Many books, articles and treatises have been written about budget preparations, and if you read many of them you will find that after about 10 minutes you are completely confused.

Confusion is only part of your problem; the largest part is actually sitting down and preparing a budget.

If you have run a household budget, you will find it is not much different from the budget you must set up to operate your hospital or department. Let us review a household budget. You have X number of dollars as income. This is after taxes and any other deductions you might have as an individual. You also have certain bills that must be paid. The major ones are for the mortgage or rent, food, heating, light, telephone, car insurance, life insurance, and hospital insurance. After these have been paid, the money that is left is allocated to entertainment, clothes, travel, vacation, and transportation, and by the time everything is added up most of us find that we are in the red, that is, we do not have enough money left to cover all the remaining expenses. We still have some bills outstanding and no money to pay them.

How To Prepare a Budget

If you are preparing a budget for your department, you have a somewhat similar situation. You must pay all the bills required to keep the hospital (or your department) operating: gas and electricity, rent or mortgage, telephone and, of course, salaries and benefits.

The budget should be divided into anticipated income and expenses. Income can be projected on the basis of patient days, services rendered per patient day, and the charges that may be made for these services.

Expenses involve personnel costs, which amount to about 70 percent of total expenses; materials; leases and contracts, and overhead costs. Overhead costs usually include interest on indebtedness, utilities, phone, building maintenance, and various other costs that cannot be allocated to a specific area. Try to keep your department's expenses within the revenue projected by the administrator or comptroller for your department.

Personnel costs are defined in large part by the salaries of permanent employees who are already working at the start of the fiscal year. Additional personnel may be anticipated (or reductions may be planned) and the adjustments must be made for their impact. Supplies can be estimated on the basis of previous experience, and equipment leases may already be in effect. If new equipment is anticipated, and changes made in supplies, etc., these can be figured into the totals already established. Any total increase in costs must be offset by a corresponding increase in income. If the increase in income that you can conservatively project does not more than offset increased costs that are estimated any change you plan should be studied very carefully.

Here is a very simple approach to preparing a budget.

Salaries

List the number of people you have working for you and how much you pay them by the hour. You have two categories of employees—those who do not punch a time clock and those who do. It is easy to figure the salaries of those who punch a clock. Those who do not are required to work 35 or 40 hours a week; however, the reason they do not punch a clock is because as professional individuals they may be called upon to travel or to work overtime or on weekends. It is to the hospital's benefit to pay them a straight salary. That is, they are paid by the week regardless of how much time they put in. It could be 35 or 40 or 75 hours, which is why these people in most instances are paid at a higher rate than is the average time-clock employee.

Overhead Costs

Once you have taken into account all the people on your staff (and be sure to include yourself), the next step is to work out the overhead costs for your unit, if you are a department head. This would include the space allocated to your operation.

How do you determine the cost of this space? First, put down the rental or mortgage cost of the total building and then break that cost down according to the cost per cubic foot. By determining the number of cubic feet your unit occupies, you can determine your share of the over-all cost. Figure the cost per month and multiply it by 12 to arrive at the yearly cost. Next, consider all the other costs (telephone, light, heat, supplies, etc.) that must be included in the total overhead and apply the same principle of breaking them down according to the percentage of the total that would be chargeable to your department. These figures can be obtained from the hospital accounting office. Usually they are allocated by the hospital for your department.

New Equipment

With these basics out of the way, you are still not out of the woods. What about purchasing new equipment? We have figured so far on old equipment, space, materials and supplies that are now being used, but suppose you wish to purchase something new. You should have a category set aside for new or needed equipment. This way you would have built into your budget items that you need or will be needing for the fiscal year. In this connection, recall that budgets are set up for a fiscal year. Some institutions prefer to go from June to June rather than from January to January. So you will have to establish your budget according to the policy of the organization. Usually, you would propose the purchase of new equipment and justify its purchase.

Staff

What about staff requirements? We figured out how much it cost us to maintain the people we have. But, suppose you propose to add some new people. Have you allocated monies for such a situation? Have you justified the need for additional personnel?

Have you figured increases in your budget? Every year there are people who feel, justifiably, that their salaries should be increased. These can be given only if you have budgeted for them. How much is it going to cost you to give everyone an increase? Most institutions set a mandatory maximum or minimum requirement for salary increases and you are allocated a percentage of the total. Let us say $1000 is available for this purpose to be divided among four departments. You would get 25 percent. You now have to dispense this money to the people who in your estimation are working the hardest or best for your operation. If you don't allocate the funds correctly some employees may quit. So keep in mind that every year a company will give X number of dollars to its managers to be disseminated to the employees under them and you must be prepared to break down this percentage to what is fair and equitable to those concerned.

Equipment

Your budget must also allow for rental or leasing of such equipment as Xerox™ copiers or other large equipment. Some of the leased equipment may be under contract and contracts come due at different times of the year. Again, money has to be allocated for this.

You may encounter the need for something for which there is no precedent and for which no policy has been issued. How do you go about allocating funds for this?

The best way is to estimate what you think you will need and indicate in your budget that it is only an estimate and that you may have to ask for additional funding because this is a situation which you do not and cannot project.

Miscellaneous

Finally, there is that all-encompassing title, "miscellaneous." In this you may include money for travel either for yourself or persons under your jurisdiction. If you entertain the possibility of traveling you should ask your supervisor to submit possible travel time before you submit your budget.

Some needs may arise for which you have not budgeted but if the over-all budget has been planned properly funds can be diverted from certain sections to others in order to balance it out. A contingency factor should be allowed as a percentage of the total budget after you have included everything you consider necessary to cover your needs for the year. One percent of your total budget should be enough to cover any problems that may come up.

How To Stay Within a Budget

Now that you have put together a budget you are faced with the problem of how to stay within it. How well you succeed is really going to depend on how well the budget was prepared. If you go into the red in certain areas, if you have budgeted correctly you should be able to divert funds from one section to cover you in another. For example, suppose you have budgeted for travel for one year the sum of $1000 but because of certain urgent problems that have come up you are required to go over that budget by $500. If you have budgeted $1000 for a new machine and there is no need to buy it you can divert $500 of this to cover the added cost of travel. Or, if under equipment rental you had anticipated renting a piece of equipment for $500 and decide you no longer need it, you can divert that fund to cover the deficit in travel.

But suppose you need everything you have projected. Everything you have taken into account is used as you expected. You now have an emergency situation: You need $500 to $1000 and there is no place to get the money. Then you are faced with the problem of having to go into the red. This may be a temporary situation in the event that your deficit will be created by the purchase of a piece of essential equipment, because in six months the income from this new equipment can more than make up for the deficit. Do not compromise by not hiring people or not getting the job done properly because you are afraid of going over the budget. If your calculations are correct and if you feel that the income from the new equipment will cover your loss, then go ahead and buy the equipment. Remember, however, to consult your supervisor before you make any final decision.

Accountability

However, you may be wrong and find that at the end of your particular budget year you are in the red. Then you are faced with the day of reckoning. You will probably be called in by your superior to review your budget for the year. If he has been lax during the year you may not have been caught until now. What he is going to ask is an accounting for the money you have spent. If during the year you have kept good records and receipts for all outlays and there is a good reason for being in the red your superior may be sympathetic. However, if your records are shabby, if you have completely mismanaged your operation and at the end of the year you are not only in the red but in such a bad situation that it will take a battery of accountants to unwind your budget, then you must be willing to take the responsibility for the problem you yourself have created.

You could perhaps have avoided some of these problems by auditing yourself at least once a month. You could have seen a dangerous trend and recognized that you were spending more and more and getting less and less return.

Waiting until the end of the year to inform your superior that you are in the red and have been since the second month of your budget is poor money accountability. Because at this day of reckoning not only do you have a problem with money accountability, you must also account for the materials and equipment for which you are responsible. These are now just as important as the money you have to account for.

Proposed Budget

There is a great deal of time and thought involved in setting up a good, workable budget. All the categories that have been discussed and many more will have to be taken into account. The unfortunate part of a budget is that when it is submitted and accepted, you are held accountable for it. So it behooves you to make a very close evaluation before you submit what you call a budget. One technique in budget preparation you can keep in mind is to submit it as a "proposed budget." You may find that the powers that be will review your budget and knock it down. It is safe to say that very few budgets are increased by people in the higher echelons of the institution. The rule usually is to cut. Keep this in mind when you are preparing to submit the final budget. Between budget preparation, managing within the budget, money accountability, and materials accountability you, as a manager, are responsible for a very important portion of your entire operation. All this can be lumped together under one interesting word called "finances."

Review Questions

1. Define overhead.

2. How do you go about setting up a budget?

3. What is a contingency factor?

4. Do rentals of equipment go into a budget?

5. What items go into the categories of "miscellaneous?"

6. What is meant by the "day of reckoning?"

7. Is a household budget similar to a hospital's budget?

The Road to Success as a Manager

How does one know when he is doing a good job as a manager? As a general rule, the people you supervise will seldom tell you that you are doing a fine job. If you are not doing so well they may mention it, and your supervisor just might bring the matter up. The comments of anyone, except your supervisor, are a rather poor indication of your success and it is very possible that you will not hear much from him. It is a good process for you to establish your own criteria for judging your work performance. These criteria must have some basis in common values so that everyone–your superior, your peers, and the community–will be satisfied and agreeable with what you judge to be success.

Levels of Success

It is difficult to set out criteria that can be applied to every circumstance but there are certain general conditions that are characteristic of a well run hospital department. After you have read the following, think how it might apply to your situation or to a job you may wish to have. The points mentioned might be thought of as a hierarchy since each criterion presented here would seem to be of a slightly higher order than the one before it.

Stability

Stability is certainly a characteristic of a well managed unit. Don't be surprised if the first months on the job are rather hectic. There are sev-

eral reasons. The people around you are not yet secure. Each person has his territorial imperative and his occasional feelings of inadequacy. He is waiting for you to upset his secure little area or discover his inadequacy. There may be resentment that he was not chosen for this job rather than you. Most people do not welcome change—especially when it is a change to something unknown. It is advisable, if possible, to go slow when starting as a new supervisor. Give people a chance to see that you are not–and do not intend to be–a threat to their security. As soon as they know you, can judge your reactions and your moods, and have some feel for your way of getting things done, they will become more willing to accept your suggestions, and, after adequate explanation, will make changes.

A young supervisor, regardless of training, is likely to have some problems. Experience and a degree of maturity are a significant asset. Poise and inner security are hard to achieve by a new supervisor when he feels he is on trial. There is a natural desire to prove one's self. Like a roller skater, it may be wise just to master standing up on the skates before you try a Figure 8. Most administrators would prefer to have a stable department than one on the move but in turmoil. Start slowly by winning the confidence of people who will depend on you. See to it that essential functions are carried on at least as well as they were before you took charge. Hard work on everyone's part, but especially on yours, is usually necessary. There are many details to learn, people to study, and plans to lay. Let everyone, your supervisors as well as those who work for you, know that you are interested in doing a good job and concerned for them. It is hard to resent someone who is really trying to help you.

When stability is achieved, work will be done in a reasonably orderly manner, persons in your department will feel comfortable working with you and secure in their jobs. Turnover among your personnel should be at a supportable level and you should no longer feel threatened with failure when someone disagrees with you.

Operational Audit

A second level of success is achieved when your unit can successfully withstand an audit or an inspection of its operation. When we think of an audit we generally think of money or accounts but we may think more generally of an audit as an analysis of the operation. Your supervisor may look into the way your activities are being conducted. Are records in order? Are services being provided as required? Are patients, doctors and other employees satisfied with the way your department runs? Can you account for property, supplies, or money which has been assigned to you? If you are responsible for funds or accounts, it is customary for an organization to hire an auditor, comptroller or accountant to review the accounts and actually audit them. At any rate, the person or persons to whom you are accountable should be able to look through your affairs at any time and find them completely in order.

Very little has been said about records. Every aspect of medical care today requires records of all sorts and it is not easy to generalize. Many types of hospital records are required and it is wise to know exactly what records you must keep, how long they must be kept, and for what purpose they are being kept. Failure to keep records as required by law or regulation is inexcusable. Other records may be for your convenience or to document the disposition of supplies, scheduling of people, or other actions. Enough records must be kept to support your position. You cannot afford to be unable to explain any important action you take. At the same time, records may become a burden to you and the department. When files or logs are started or forms are initiated, some decision should be made about disposition of the accumulated records. Do not continue to use valuable space to store records after they have exceeded their usefulness. Occasionally, all records and correspondence should be reviewed and those that are not needed should be eliminated.

Profitability

Once the organization is able to withstand an audit of its methods of operation, the manager can begin to think about the profitability of the operation. Only a few of a hospital's departments can think about profit in terms of making money. All can think about the advantages or profits for the hospital that can be credited to them. These profits may be tangible services, such as linens washed, meals served, or treatments rendered. For some departments, the improvement in medical records, better telephone communications, or faster, neater typing may be harder to count or measure. In your particular specialty, however, you can judge whether the service you render has improved the care of the patients, service to doctors, financial status of the hospital, satisfaction of employees, etc. If your responsibility has been discharged well, you should be able to define your service in terms of profitability or advantage and the measure of this is one measure of your success.

Accreditation

Most of the areas of specialization in medical care have some form of accreditation. The process of accreditation is primarily a voluntary effort to evaluate and certify excellence in a particular pursuit. Accreditation may be awarded to an individual when he meets certain prescribed educational and practical requirements. It may also be awarded to an institution or service unit when it meets certain requirements. People and departments may function quite satisfactorily without accreditation, but this mark of approval gives the public a basis for judging competence. The basis for accreditation is generally defined and the accreditation is awarded by a peer group, such as the appropriate professional organization. Such accreditation is given favorable recognition by other groups and by the general public and, in many cases, it becomes adequate proof of excellence to satisfy legal requirements such as licensure. Large insurance companies, such as Blue Cross, may recognize accreditation as a reasonable basis for deciding if a service is adequate.

When a service department or an appreciable number of people in the group are accredited by a peer group, one would be justified in feeling that it was reasonably successful.

Quality Control

It is quite possible that your department could be successful according to the tests we have discussed but still be rendering service of dubious value. Most operations now attempt some measure of quality control to test whether certain standards of operation are met. Central services may use such measures to judge whether surgical packs are properly prepared and sterilized, for example. The dietary department may use quality control to be sure meals of good quality are getting to the patient in an appetizing condition. The laboratory may need quality control to test the accuracy of its analyses, and the laundry may need to know the neatness and cleanliness of linen processed.

Quality control, like paper work, can easily become a matter of form. Measures are initiated to serve a good and useful purpose but, as time goes on, the form is carried on but the value of the procedure is lost. Quality control measures need to be changed often. New parameters of service need to be measured and new approaches tried. It is not unusual for people to change work habits to satisfy a fixed quality control check without improving the actual quality of their performance. If dishes are to be sterilized at a given temperature, for example, the thermometer is simply moved about until a spot is found where the water is hot enough to meet the requirement. This point could be 3 feet from the nearest dish. Remember, if quality control does not help you attain a higher quality of performance it is not worth the cost in time and money. Meeting high standards of quality control is a measure of your success.

Recognition

If you have achieved stability, put your affairs in an auditable condition, proved the worth of your activities, become accredited, and instituted some effective quality control and have maintained all of these for some time, the chances are good that you have gained acceptance in your hospital and community. This is a satisfying measure of success. How widely and how well you are recognized will depend on many things. Some jobs lend themselves to recognition. Others are colorless and attract little attention. Some jobs are quite difficult to perform without alienating someone. The very necessary collections department in a hospital, for example, must constantly push reluctant customers to pay their hospital bills.

Public Relations

Often it may be expedient to spend a little time on public relations. It is always easier to do business with people who like and appreciate your efforts. There are few situations where patient funds should be expended to promote the popularity of a department, of course. The direction of such efforts should be to present the efforts of your department in such a way as to improve the stature of the service you perform. Patients have a right to feel that the care they are getting is the very best that is available. When the people in your department do a good job, they should get recognition for it. The general public should learn that this group of people do a good job and that a patient is in good hands when they are on the job. Such publicity must not seem blatant or offensive and, in no case, should anyone else be made to look bad so your department will look good. Remember that recognition is one of the basic needs cited by Maslow and you are helping your employee satisfy a need in a constructive way when you help publicize his good work. The morale of the department will improve and the standard of performance will move higher. Incidentally, your success as a manager will be enhanced and you may also enjoy some recognition. Exercise care to stay out of the center of the publicity you have promoted, however.

Attaining Goals

A further measure of your success will be in your personal satisfaction with the job you have done. You may feel some measure of success as you achieve various goals along the way but you will have an especially rich feeling of personal reward when you can look about you and feel that things are running smoothly and efficiently and that your department is recognized as good. There is, of course, something in the personality of most managers that strives for perfection and always sees unfinished tasks. Still, in quiet moments they see their accomplishments in perspective and are pleased.

Most managers are competitive people who aggressively strive to reach goals. Most of us set up such goals and establish some sort of time table for reaching them. The achievement of our goals is, of course, a prime measure of the success of our venture in management. The measure of each of us as an individual can be found in our goals.

We identify with the image of the person we aspire to be and, as time goes on, we gradually become that person. If we are satisfied with mediocre aims, the goal we reach will probably be mediocre. Writers have stressed the point continually. "Not failure, but low aim, is crime," is an oft quoted expression. We have been so vaccinated with such expressions that we are nearly immune to the philosophy they espouse. Think for a moment about the fact that you will almost certainly never rise higher than the goals you set for yourself and reflect on what such success will mean to you.

Possibly the ultimate in success of your efforts as manager is a sense of security. When you have become successful in all of the ways we have discussed, you will be recognized as valuable to the organization and little consideration is likely to be given to replacing you. Your peers will accept the fact that you are able to help them grow and develop. You will probably have found new, higher goals and found that satisfaction is not in achieving a goal but in striving for it.

Responsibilities

When you accept the task of managing a group, you also accept certain responsibilities. Many of these are clearly implied. You are responsible for the space, material and equipment provided to you. You accept the responsibility for achieving the objective of the group you manage, whether it is cleaning floors or posting patients' bills. Other responsibilities are possibly a little less obvious. You accept the responsibility for job assignments, classification and pay of workers, but you should also feel some sense of responsibility for them as individuals. On your shoulders in large part will ride the satisfaction, enjoyment, frustrations and defeats of each individual. His learning and progress, financial security and standard of living will depend upon his success under your leadership. Your decisions need to be more deliberate and better thought out because of this special responsibility for the welfare of those who work for you.

Another responsibility that is not so apparent is the responsibility to protect the organization's good name and reputation. Most of us soon begin to feel that any criticism of our institution is an attack on us personally since the efforts which we have put forth have had something to do with making it what it is. Some supervisors do not get this sense of identification and are able to go along criticizing their superior's decisions and undermining the effectiveness of their hospitals. The same people probably would insist on their right to smoke in a dynamite factory. When you are put in a position of authority, your supervisor has complimented you and given you something of value (aside from the money you'll be getting to do a good job). It is in extremely poor taste to repay this with disloyalty but it also shows poor judgment. One gets a mental picture of a person sitting on a limb, happily sawing it off close to the tree trunk.

Hospitals in particular are subject to liability suits by patients who have suffered real or imagined loss, pain and suffering or inconvenience. As a manager, it is your job to see that the patient has no reason to bring action against the hospital. This may be done in various ways. Obviously, if patient care is rendered in the way it should be, there is less opportunity for legal suits. In practice, however, more such suits are brought by people who have suffered slights and insults than by people who have suffered actual injury. That is to say, the person who is pleased with the care he receives is much less likely to attack the hospital and doctor than the one who feels offended, slighted, or ignored. Almost always, patient complaints can be traced to an employee who has handled an interpersonal situation poorly. Either the attitude of such an employee is basically poor or his training and indoctrination have been badly neglected.

Another large responsibility of the manager is the safety of his group and of the hospital in general. Hospital accidents and fires can be real disasters. Fire codes are strict and fire plans are quite detailed. All safety regulations and codes should be followed meticulously and constant vigilance is needed. Fires, explosions, chemical poisonings, equipment failures, accidents on wet floors, falls and infections are all largely preventable. The supervisor has a responsibility to do his best to avoid all of these through careful attention and planning.

You represent a member of your peer group— a technician, a nurse, a secretary, a therapist— who has been given a chance to prove that you have the stuff to succeed. You are forever an example of your kind who was given a chance to move up and you have a responsibility to those who may follow up the ladder. If you fail to do your best, the next representative of your group may never get the chance to try.

Review Questions

1. At the present time, what accomplishments would make you feel you had succeeded?

2. What general responsibilities does a manager have?

3. Write a brief fire plan for the building you are in now. What does the person who discovered the fire do? How are people evacuated? Who has responsibilities of helping? Who is in charge?

4. Write a brief statement concerning your goals and how you plan to work toward them. Will achieving these goals bring about the feeling of success described in this chapter?

5. For your own future use, prepare a code of ethics that you feel will help you as you progress to greater responsibilities.

Recommended Reading

Ardrey, Robert: *The Territorial Imperative*. New York: Atheneum Publishers, 1966.

Argyris, C.: *Personality and Organization*. New York: Harper & Bros., 1957.

Babcock, M.D. (Quoted by Reinhard Bendix): *Work and Authority in Industry*. New York: John Wiley and Sons, 1956.

Dunnette, M., and Kirchner, W.K.: *Psychology Applied to Industry*. New York: Appleton-Century Crofts, 1965.

Fowler, H.: *Curiosity and Exploratory Behavior*. New York: Macmillan Company, 1965.

Herzberg, Frederick: *Work and the Nature of Man*. Cleveland and New York: The World Publishing Company, 1969.

Herzberg, Frederick, et al: *The Motivation to Work*. New York: John Wiley and Sons, 1959.

Heyel, Carl: *Management for Modern Supervisors*. New York: American Management Association.

Killian, Ray A.: *Managers Must Lead*. New York: American Management Association.

Leadership on the Job—Guides to Good Supervision. New York: American Management Association.

Maslow, Abraham H.: *A Theory for Human Motivation*. Psychological Review, 50:370-396 (July) 1943.

NOTES

NOTES

NOTES

Index

Computers, 59
  hospital applications, 63
  how computer works, 60
  laboratory-based system, 66
  management applications, 66
  patient records, 59

Employees, 24, 33
  how to find, 24
  how to train, 28
  see also Personnel

Finances, 90
  budget, 90
    accountability, 91
    equipment, 91
    overhead costs, 91
    salaries, 91
    staff, 91

Health care system, 9

Hospitals and employees, 12
  career in hospital work, 14
  major departments, 12

Leasing, 79

Manager, road to success, 95
  level of success, 95
    accreditation, 96
    attaining goals, 97
    operational audit, 96
    profitability, 96
    public relations, 97
    quality control, 96
    recognition, 97
  responsibilities, 98

Personnel supervision, 24
  hiring employees, 24
    interviews, 26
  interpersonal relations, 33
    challenge to authority, 43
    communications, 36
    employee characteristics, 34
    human needs and motivations, 45
    territorial imperative, 41
  training employees, 28
  orientation, 28
  policies, 28

Physical resources, 70
  care of equipment, 71
  inventory, 71
  obsolescence and deterioration, 75
    records of equipment repair, 76
  repair and maintenance, 70
  space arrangement, 70

Purchasing and leasing, 79
  cost analysis, 82
  equipment leasing, 79
  glossary of terms, 86
  purchasing, 85

Staffing, 52

Supervision, 24

Work organization, 52
  evaluations, 56
  job descriptions, 55
  organizational plan, 52
  procedure manuals, 56